Self-Assess~ of

Small Animal Soft Tissue Surgery

Stephen D. Gilson
DVM, Dipl ACVS
Sōnōra Veterinary Surgery and Oncology
Scottsdale, Arizona, USA

Manson Publishing/The Veterinary Press

Copyright © 1998 Manson Publishing Ltd
ISBN: 1-874545-64-2

A CIP catalogue record for this book is available from the British Library.

For full details of all Manson Publishing Ltd titles please write to:
Manson Publishing Ltd, 73 Corringham Road, London NW11 7DL.

Text editing: Peter Beynon
Typesetting, design and layout: Paul Bennett
Colour reproduction: Tenon & Polert Colour Scanning Ltd., Hong Kong
Printed by: Grafos S.A., Barcelona, Spain

Preface

This title provides a brief but broad overview of all aspects of general surgery for small animals. Like other titles in the *Self-Assessment Colour Review* series, the questions are divided into multiple parts and most are accompanied by an illustration, diagnostic image or clinical photograph. The answers are of moderate length and are designed to provide the reader with specific considerations for the management of the disease process presented. The content and format of the cases are presented in a manner akin to clinical experience, and will appeal equally to veterinary students, practitioners with an interest in surgery and surgeons in training. They also provide a spectrum of challenge ranging from simple to difficult, with most of the questions being moderately difficult.

The cases were provided by an international group of authors. Surgery is an inherently controversial topic, so the reader may find variations to the diagnostic and treatment recommendations with which they are familiar. I have attempted to dampen points of controversy, but ask the reader to consider some of the different approaches presented herein with an open mind.

This text is the culmination of many hours of work, and my hope is that you enjoy the book and that you are surgically more learned having read it.

Stephen D. Gilson
1997

Contributors

Ana Mayenco Aguirre, DVM
Universidad Complutense de Madrid,
Madrid, Spain

Fidel SanRomán Ascaso, DVM, DDS, MD
Universidad Complutense de Madrid,
Madrid, Spain

R. Avery Bennett, DVM, MS, Dipl ACVS
University of Florida, Gainesville, Florida,
USA

Bernard Bouvy, DVM, MSc, Dipl ACVS
& ECVS
Clinique Vétérinaire Frégis, Arcueil,
France

Phyllis Ann Ciekot, DVM, MS, Dipl
ACVIM (Oncology)
Sonora Veterinary Surgery and Oncology,
Scottsdale, Arizona, USA

Gilles Dupré, DVM, Dipl ECVS
Clinique Vétérinaire Frégis, Arcueil, France

Paloma García Fernández, DVM
Universidad Complutense de Madrid,
Madrid, Spain

Stephen D. Gilson, DVM, Dipl ACVS
Sonora Veterinary Surgery and Oncology,
Scottsdale, Arizona, USA

Joseph Harari, DVM, MS, Dipl ACVS
Rowley Memorial Animal Hospital,
Springfield, Massachusetts, USA

Elizabeth M. Hardie, DVM, PhD,
Dipl ACVS
North Carolina State University, Raleigh,
North Carolina, USA

Dudley E. Johnston, BVSc, MVSc, AM,
Dipl ACVS & ECVS
Hebrew University of Jerusalem, Rehovot,
Israel

Jolle Kirpensteijn, DVM, MS, Dipl
ACVS & ECVS
University of Utrecht, Utrecht,
The Netherlands

Mercedes Sánchez de la Muela, DVM
Universidad Complutense de Madrid,
Madrid, Spain

Maura G. O'Brien, DVM, Dipl ACVS
VCA West Los Angeles Animal Hospital,
Los Angeles, California, USA

Debora J. Osuna, BS, DVM, Dipl ACVS
Franklin Veterinary Services Referral
Centre, Papakura, New Zealand

Pilar Llorens Pena, MD
Universidad Complutense de Madrid,
Madrid, Spain

Betina C. Rama, DVM
Iams Company, Buenos Aires, Argentina

Leonardo J. Sepiurka, DVM
College of Veterinary Medicine, Buenos
Aires, Argentina

Nick Sharp, BVetMed, PhD, Dipl ACVS,
ACVIM & ECVS, MRCVS
North Carolina State University, Raleigh,
North Carolina, USA

Mark M. Smith, VMD, Dipl ACVS
Virginia–Maryland Regional College of
Veterinary Medicine, Blacksburg,
Virginia, USA

Mark J. Soderstrom, DVM
Oklahoma State University, Stillwater,
Oklahoma, USA

Jesús Rodríguez Quiros, DVM
Universidad Complutense de Madrid,
Madrid, Spain

Sharon Ullman, DVM, Dipl ACVS
Veterinary Surgical Associates, Concord,
California, USA

Katherine Wells, DVM
Metroplex Veterinary Center, Irving,
Texas, USA

C.D. van Zuilen, DVM
University of Utrecht, Utrecht,
The Netherlands

Acknowledgements

I would first and foremost like to thank the international group of contributing authors and the staff at Manson Publishing for their outstanding and timely efforts – I realize it was often a challenge collaborating with an overworked editor in a different time zone. Without the co-authors I could not have assembled a text with this quality of content; and without the organizational skills, guidance and persistent prodding of Jonathan Gregory, Clair Chaventré and Paul Bennett at Manson Publishing I could not have assembled it in this century!

On a broader scale I want to give long overdue thanks to my friends and colleagues: Don Morshead for providing the spark that began my interest in surgery; Peter Schwarz who encouraged and guided me through my internship; and long-time friend and mentor Elizabeth Stone who, in addition to providing several of the photographs used in the text, has had the greatest impact on my professional development. Thanks also to the many other people I owe for my training and advancement as a surgeon – you know who you are and more importantly I know who you are.

The following gave their permission for the following figures to be reproduced in the book (identified by question numbers):

13 Courtesy of Mary Mahaffey, DVM, MS, Dipl ACVR

28b Reproduced with permission from Smith, M.M. and Waldron, D.R. (1993) Approach to the hard palate. In: *Atlas of Approaches for General Surgery of the Dog and Cat*. Eds Smith, M.M. and Waldron, D.R. WB Saunders, Philadelphia, pp.72–73.

168a–c, 176a, b, 192, 209a Copyright © 1988, United States Surgical Corporation. All rights reserved. Reprinted with the permission of the United States Surgical Corporation.

172 Reprinted with permission of the *Journal of the American Animal Hospitals Association*.

Abbreviations

AGID	Agar gel immunodiffusion	HCG	Human chorionic gonadotrophin
bpm	Beats per minute	i/m	Intramuscular
BUN	Blood urea nitrogen	i/v	Intravenous
CBC	Complete blood count	LH	Luteinizing hormone
ECG	Electrocardiogram	MIC	Minimum inhibitory concentration
ELISA	Enzyme-linked immunosorbent assay	PCV	Packed cell volume
FeLV	Feline leukemia virus	p/o	*Per os* (by mouth)
FIV	Feline immunodeficiency virus	q	Every
GnRH	Gonadotrophin-releasing hormone	s/c	Subcutaneous
		tid	*Ter in die* (three times a day)

Classification of cases

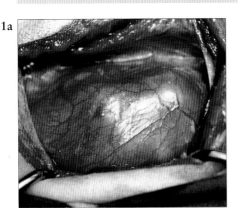
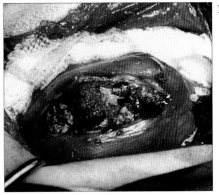

1 A six-month-old Cairn Terrier is presented for acute onset of drooling, regurgitation, anorexia and cervical pain. An esophageal foreign body is detected by plain radiography of the cervical region.
i. Name common locations for esophageal foreign body entrapment.
ii. Describe some non-surgical alternatives and list the advantages of these methods.
iii. Name several indications for surgical intervention.
iv. Describe the surgical procedure shown (1a, b).

2 A surgical procedure underway in the oral cavity of a four-month-old, male Bulldog is shown (2). The owner's complaint is that the dog has a chronic mucopurulent nasal discharge, coughs when eating or drinking, and has not been gaining weight at a rate equal to that of his litter mates. He also has a foul odor from the oral cavity.
i. What is the diagnosis?
ii. What secondary complication may be associated with this defect?
iii. What are three principles to be followed during surgical repair of this problem?

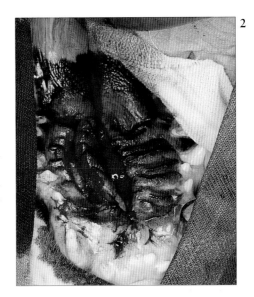

3 Describe four ways tissues can be cut/incised. What are the advantages and disadvantages of each?

1 i. Foreign body entrapment caused by limited ability of the esophagus to dilate at certain locations is most common at the pharynx, thoracic inlet, base of the heart and just before the cardia.
ii. Non-surgical management consists of foreign body retrieval by forceps under guidance of a rigid or flexible endoscope, or by the Foley catheter technique. Non-surgical removal of foreign bodies results in lower morbidity and shortens hospitalization in uncomplicated cases. A recovery rate of 98% is reported after foreign body removal without surgery.
iii. Conservative treatment is attempted prior to surgery, except when there is evidence of esophageal perforation, large areas of necrotic tissue, or immobility of the foreign body. Clean lacerations that do not extend through the full thickness of the esophageal wall may be left to heal secondarily. Endoscopy allows direct visualization of the foreign body and esophageal mucosa.
iv. Cervical esophagotomy. The esophagus is visualized beside the trachea after a ventral midline skin incision and separation of the sternohyoideus and sternothyroideus muscles. The esophagus is incised longitudinally and the foreign body removed. Closure of the esophagus is by simple interrupted suture in the mucosa and submucosa, followed by a second interrupted layer in the muscularis adventitia.

2 i. Congenital cleft of the hard and soft palates (secondary palatal defect).
ii. Aspiration pneumonia is often a complication of secondary palate defects. The animal should be evaluated with thoracic radiographs and treated appropriately prior to surgical correction of the palate defect.
iii. Repair flaps should be larger than the primary defect to reduce tension on suture lines. Connective tissue and vascular supply is preserved by limited meticulous dissection (avoid the palatine artery) and gentle tissue handling. Tissue flaps are apposed to cleanly incised epithelium to ensure healing. Temporary feeding via a pharyngostomy or gastrostomy tube should be considered to bypass the oral cavity during wound healing (see also **190**).

3

	Advantages	Disadvantages
1. Scalpel blade	Cheap, least traumatic, good for dense tissue and tissue under tension. Gold- standard for tissue incision	Poor for loose tissues, no hemostasis, difficult to use for fine dissection around vessels and nerves
2. Electroscalpel	Decreased blood loss (coagulation), decreased foreign material (ligature), decreased operating time	Variable thermal necrosis at wound edges, delayed wound healing, decreased resistance to infection
3. Scissors	Good for loose tissues, provides some hemostasis by crushing, good depth control for cutting and dissection	Crushing damage to tissue, difficult to use in dense tissue
4. Laser	Less thermal injury than electroscalpel, resulting in decreased postoperative edema, drainage and pain; provides no-touch technique and precise tissue vaporization for meticulous dissection	High equipment cost and maintenance, delayed wound healing from thermal injury; requires special training and safety measures

4 A lateral abdominal radiograph of a three-month-old, female cat is shown (4). The animal was born with a swelling in the umbilical region that is easily reduced manually.
i. What is your diagnosis?
ii. Do you need any other tests to confirm the diagnosis?
iii. What is the treatment of choice?

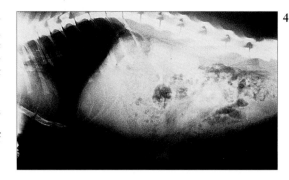

5 An eight-year-old St. Bernard is presented with signs of depression, abdominal distension and non-productive vomiting (5).
i. What is the most likely diagnosis?
ii. Describe the initial presurgical therapy.
ii. Describe the surgical correction of the problem, and name different surgical techniques to prevent recurrence.

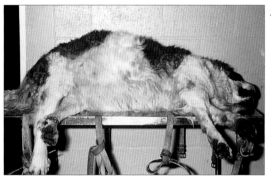

6 A five-week-old, female Brittany Spaniel puppy is presented for two day duration of anorexia, vomiting and depression. The owner suspects the puppy may have swallowed a small plastic toy. On examination, the puppy's temperature is 37.2°C, heart rate is 150 bpm and pulses are weak.
i. How is hydration status best assessed in puppies less than six weeks of age?
ii. You have assessed the puppy to be severely dehydrated. By what routes can fluid therapy be administered?
iii. The abdomen is slightly distended and painful to palpation. Abdominal radiographs indicate there is an intestinal obstruction and a moderate amount of peritoneal effusion. Relevant hemogram and serum chemistry values are: PCV 0.6 l/l (60%); serum protein 75 g/l (7.5 g/dl); glucose 2.5 mmol/l (45 mg/dl); urea 6.64 mmol/l (BUN 40 mg/dl); potassium 3.0 mmol/l (3.0 mEq/l). Exploratory laparotomy is planned to treat the gastrointestinal obstruction. What replacement fluids are used to rehydrate this puppy? What considerations are made prior to administration? What rate of administration is appropriate? How is overhydration prevented?

4 i. A congenital umbilical hernia containing omentum and small intestine.

ii. In this case it is not necessary to perform other diagnostic tests. The radiographs show air-filled tubular structures, typical of small intestinal loops, outside the abdominal wall. In other less obvious cases it may be useful to perform a barium study or, if the presence of a herniated parenchymatous organ (e.g. liver, spleen) is suspected, then sonography can be used.

iii. Treatment is by surgical reduction of the hernial contents and suturing closed the defect edges. Due to the size of this particular hernia, it is not recommended to wait for spontaneous resolution; small hernias will often be harmlessly occluded by falciform ligament or omentum. Larger hernias present the risk of bowel obstruction or visceral organ strangulation and are best repaired by early surgery.

5 i. Gastric dilatation-volvulus.

ii. Initial treatment consists of gastric decompression and treatment of shock. Gastric decompression is achieved by passing a stomach tube, percutaneous needle trocarization or temporary gastrostomy.

iii. A standard midline laparotomy is performed and the stomach is repositioned and decompressed. Stomach contents are removed using a large stomach tube or through a gastrotomy incision. The viability of the stomach is evaluated and non-viable parts are resected. The spleen is repositioned and inspected. Splenectomy is performed if viability is in doubt. The stomach is secured in a normal position by attaching the pyloric antral region to the adjacent right abdominal wall. Gastropexy techniques include tube gastrostomy and circumcostal, belt loop and incision gastropexy.

6 i. In animals younger than six weeks of age, use of skin turgor is not accurate to estimate dehydration. Evaluation of mucous membrane moistness and urine color are more accurate. The urine of puppies at this age should be clear and colorless. Any color tinting indicates dehydration.

ii. In very young animals, fluids can be administered i/v through the jugular or cephalic veins, and intraosseously into the long bones. An intraosseous needle can be readily placed in the femur, tibia, humerus or ulna. Flow rates of up to 11 ml/min can be achieved with gravity flow through an intraosseous catheter.

iii. A replacement fluid such as Ringer's solution with 5% dextrose is utilized best by young animals. To treat acute hypoglycemia, replace glucose with 1–2 ml/kg of 10–25% dextrose solution; maintain plasma glucose concentration at 4.5–11.2 mmol/l (80–200 mg/dl). Fluids are warmed prior to administration, and potassium chloride is added if serum potassium concentration is less than 2.5 mmol/l (2.5 mEq/l). A basal fluid administration rate of 10–20 ml/kg/hour is recommended during anesthesia to prevent hypovolemia and maintain renal perfusion. To prevent overhydration, regularly assess for cardiopulmonary abnormalities such as tachypnea, dyspnea and cough. Weigh animals 3–4 times daily to monitor weight gain. Chemosis, exophthalmos and restlessness are other signs of overhydration.

7 A four-year-old cat is diagnosed with hypertrophic cardiomyopathy.
i. What is a common vascular complication associated with this disease process?
ii. What are three commonly noted clinical or physical examination findings associated with this condition?
iii. Is surgery useful for treatment?
iv. What is the prognosis?

8 i. Identify this instrument (8).
ii. What is its use?
iii. What are some examples of alternative instruments?

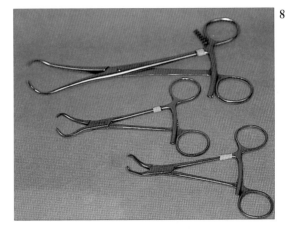

9 An exploratory laparotomy is performed on a six-year-old dog with peracute signs of depression and hematochezia (9).
i. What is the diagnosis?
ii. What breed is presumably predisposed, and what is the prognosis?
iii. What disease syndrome may ensue after resection of more than 70–80% of the small intestine? Give the most common clinical signs of this syndrome and what therapy should be instituted.

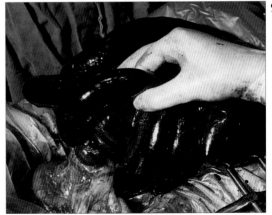

7 i. Aortic thromboembolism. Thromboemboli commonly lodge at the aortic trifurcation and extended into the branches. Peripheral thromboemboli may originate from cardiac thrombi which dislodge and pass into the aorta. Occasionally, cardiac thrombi are detected using ultrasound.
ii. Common abnormalities include paraparesis, pain, hypothermia and ischemia of the hindlimbs; and auscultation of a murmur, gallop sound or arrhythmia. Absent or weak femoral pulses indicate presence of a thrombus. Dyspnea and tachypnea may also be observed.
iii. Treatment includes supportive therapy with fluids and diuretics, use of a vasodilator such as acepromazine, and an anticoagulant such as heparin, aspirin, or warfarin. Heparin is generally used in the acute phase, and warfarin for long-term anticoagulant therapy. Clot dissolution has been achieved using streptokinase and urokinase.
Surgical removal of aortic thromboemboli has not been rewarding. It is best performed within four hours of embolization. Amputation of the left atrial appendage has also been suggested to eliminate the nidus for thrombus formation. In most cases, surgery is not rewarding and medical management is preferred.
iv. A recent study showed that affected cats had a 34% chance of surviving the initial thromboembolic episode; those that did had an average survival of 11.5 months. Re-embolization was common. Prognosis varies with the severity of the embolic event, degree of ischemia, evidence of abdominal organ infarction and severity of the underlying cardiac disease.

8 i. Pointed bone reduction forceps.
ii. Maintenance of reduction during fixation of fractured bones.
iii. Richard's and Verbrugge bone holding forceps are used for maintaining reduction or manipulation of fragments. These forceps are usually restricted to use on tubular bones because of their shape.

9 i. Mesenteric volvulus.
ii. German Shepherd Dog. The prognosis of mesenteric volvulus is extremely poor because of the peracute nature of the disease and the rapid total occlusion of blood supply to a large part of the intestinal tract.
iii. Short bowel syndrome. The most common clinical signs include chronic diarrhea, steatorrhea, weight loss and malnutrition. Medical therapy consists of feeding multiple small meals per day of a fat-restricted diet, oral antibiotics for bacterial overgrowth, cimetidine for gastric hypersecretion and vitamin supplementation.

10 With many types of sutures currently available, proper selection may be difficult. Certain principles are considered when choosing a suture material.
i. How strong should sutures be and, ideally, how rapidly should they lose strength while being absorbed?
ii. Can suture materials enhance a wound's ability to resist infection?

11a 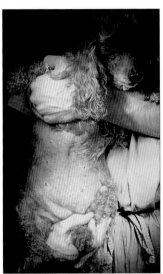 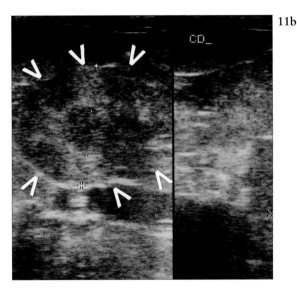 11b

11 An 11-year-old, spayed female Poodle (**11a**) presented with a history of polyuria and polydipsia, bilaterally symmetrical alopecia and a pot-bellied, pendulous abdomen. A diagnosis of hyperadrenocorticism was made after performing the following tests: CBC, serum chemistry profile, urinalysis, ACTH stimulation test and high-dose dexamethasone suppression test. Abdominal radiography and ultrasonography were used to examine the adrenal glands. An enlarged left adrenal gland (**11b**, arrowed) was found. The right adrenal gland could not be visualized. A unilateral adrenal tumor was suspected as the cause of hyperadrenocorticism in this patient.
i. What treatment options are available for this condition? What are the mechanisms of action of medical treatments? What are the benefits and disadvantages of these treatments?
ii. What are some anesthetic and surgical considerations in performing adrenalectomy for an adrenal tumor?

13

10 i. Sutures should be at least as strong as the normal tissue through which they are placed. The relative rates at which sutures lose strength and the wound gains strength should be compatible. The mechanical properties of sutures should closely match those of the tissue to be closed.

ii. No, sutures potentiate wound infection. The ability of sutured tissue to resist infection varies, depending on the physical and chemical configuration of the suture. However, even the least reactive suture material will impair a wound's ability to resist infection. The ability of a suture material to potentiate acute infection appears to parallel the inflammatory response caused by that suture. Wound infections usually begin around suture materials left in the wound. Therefore, suture use should be minimized in contaminated wounds. Monofilament sutures withstand contamination better than multifilament sutures of the same material. Synthetic sutures are superior to natural sutures. Polyglycolic acid, polyglactin 910, monofilament nylon and polypropylene have the lowest incidence of infection when used in contaminated tissues.

11 i. Surgical exploratory and adrenalectomy is preferred to treat non-invasive adrenal tumors; however, it is not without risk. In one report, more than 50% of patients undergoing adrenalectomy died of complications (e.g. thromboembolism, renal failure and infection), or were euthanized due to metastatic disease at the time of surgery. Patients with adrenal adenomas had a significantly greater chance of surviving than did dogs with adenocarcinomas.

Mitotane (op'-DDD) is cytotoxic to the cortisol producing layers of the adrenal cortex; the zona fasciculata and the zona reticularis. It is a more effective therapy for treating pituitary dependent hyperadrenocorticism than for adrenal cortical tumors, but at higher doses (50–150 mg/kg daily) some response is reported for both adrenal adenomas and adenocarcinomas.

Ketoconazole administration inhibits cholesterol synthesis and blocks cortisol formation. It is safer than mitotane since it is not cytotoxic to adrenal cortical cells, but because it does not destroy the cortisol secreting cells it must be administered for life. It was shown to have better efficacy in treating adrenal dependent hyperadrenocorticism as compared to mitotane.

ii. Hyperadrenocorticism can result in fluid and electrolyte imbalances, infection, poor wound healing, pancreatitis and thromboembolic disease. All fluid and electrolyte imbalances are corrected prior to anesthesia. Antibiotics are administered in the perioperative period and the surgeon should rigidly adhere to principles of aseptic surgery. Some surgeons feel that due to poor wound healing and muscle atrophy in these patients, a flank laparotomy may be a better surgical approach to the affected adrenal gland. Although the latter does not provide exposure to the entire abdominal cavity, the flank incision is subject to less tension than a ventral abdominal incision. Adrenalectomy may result in sudden decrease of serum cortisol levels and corticosteroids are administered perioperatively to avoid an acute Addisonian crisis.

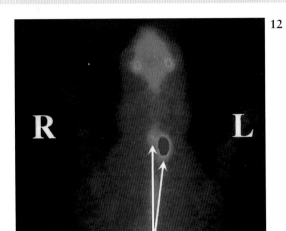

12 A 13-year-old, castrated male cat was presented with a history of weight loss despite a ravenous appetite. A cervical nodule was palpated during physical examination. Hyperthyroidism is a differential diagnosis in this patient. It is now becoming more commonplace to diagnose and treat hyperthyroidism in its early stages prior to development of these classic symptoms.

i. What diagnostic test is represented (12, thyroid adenomas arrowed)?

ii. What other diagnostic tests are reported to help diagnose occult or early hyperthyroidism?

iii. What other concurrent conditions are frequently present in cats diagnosed with hyperthyroidism?

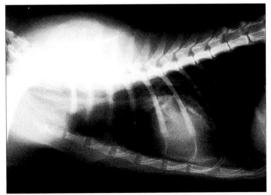

13 You are presented with a cat in severe respiratory distress. The cat was hit by a car two weeks previously and was treated by an emergency clinic. Because chest trauma was present, thoracic radiographs are made (13).

i. Based on the radiograph, what is your diagnosis?

ii. Describe how this injury occurs.

iii. Does this cat most likely have inspiratory or expiratory dyspnea, and why?

iv. Describe the surgical management of this problem.

12 i. Radionuclide imaging. Radioactive technetium-99m is administered intravenously and the neck is scanned by gamma camera. All secretory glands take up the radioactive material and in the normal patient thyroid glands show the same degree of reactivity as salivary glands. Hyperfunctioning thyroid glands show increased uptake. Radionuclide imaging also detects metastatic and ectopic lesions.

ii. Serum concentrations of thyroxine (T4) and triiodothyronine (T3) may be elevated; increased T4 concentrations are more reliable for diagnosing hyperthyroidism.

T3 suppression test – serum T3 and T4 concentrations are determined before and after T3 (oral preparation: liothyronine) is administered for three days. In normal cats T4 concentrations decrease markedly; in cats with hyperthyroidism the glands function autonomously and are not responsive to negative feedback of the thyroid hormone axis, therefore suppression of T4 is minimal.

Thyrotropin-releasing hormone (TRH) stimulation test – serum T4 concentration is measured before and after administration of exogenous thyrotropin releasing agent. In normal cats T4 concentration increases; in hyperthyroid cats T4 concentrations stay the same or only increase slightly. This test is not yet widely available and needs further study.

iii. Hypertrophic cardiomyopathy is a common sequela of hyperthyroidism. Cardiac changes induced are reversible in the majority of cats successfully treated for hyperthyroidism. Other common concurrent conditions of older hyperthyroid cats include chronic renal disease and hepatopathies.

13 i. Tracheal avulsion, rupture or transection are terms used to describe this condition. The intrathoracic trachea is transected.

ii. The trachea is rapidly and severely stretched. The carina and lungs are fixed in their location and as the trachea is stretched, it tears just cranial to the carina. Tissues surrounding the trachea usually do not tear and pneumothorax does not occur. As healing progresses and scar tissue matures, stenosis or displacement of the trachea result in respiratory distress.

iii. Expiratory dyspnea is most prominent, because as the patient exhales, intrathoracic pressure increases and tends to collapse the pseudotrachea formed around the defect. During inspiration, there is negative intrathoracic pressure which tends to open this area.

iv. The challenge for surgery is to maintain anesthesia and controlled ventilation during thoracotomy. The endotracheal tube must be long enough to reach the carina. It is wise to have a sterile endotracheal tube and breathing circuit which can be placed into the aboral portion of the trachea once the thoracotomy is performed. A right, 4th intercostal lateral thoracotomy is made. The azygous vein may need to be ligated for adequate exposure. The defect is identified and, if possible, the endotracheal tube placed *per os* is guided into the aboral segment. If the tube cannot be quickly advanced into the aboral segment, the pseudotracheal tissue is incised and a sterile endotracheal tube is inserted and connected to a sterile breathing circuit. The pseudotrachea is excised and the trachea prepared for anastomosis. The *per os* endotracheal tube is now advanced into the aboral segment and the trachea anastomosed in a routine manner. After anastomosis, if there is a leak, a mediastinal pleural patch is sutured around the anastomosis to provide adequate seal.

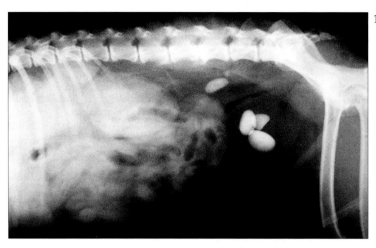

14a

14 A lateral radiograph of a ten-year-old Miniature Schnauzer presented with a history of anorexia, lethargy and dysuria for three days is shown (**14a**). On physical examination the dog was depressed, lethargic and febrile (39.4°C/103°F). It had a history of chronic urolithiasis and had undergone two cystotomies, and prescrotal urethrostomy in the past three years.
i. Give your diagnosis.
ii. What diagnostic tests would you consider before taking this dog to surgery?
iii. What are treatment options for this disease?
iv. To perform ureterotomy for calculus removal, would you incise the ureter proximal or distal to the calculus, and which suture material would you use to close the incision? Would you temporarily stent the ureter?

15 This is a wound complication that occurred four days after surgery for osteochondritis dissecans of the humeral head (**15**).
i. What is the complication and the basis for its occurrence?
ii. How does this lesion affect wound healing?
iii. What are treatment options and prognosis?

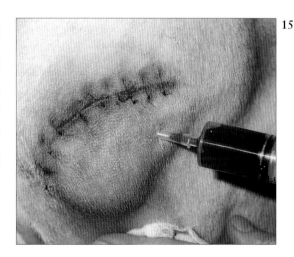

15

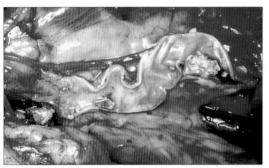

14b

14 i. A ureteral calculus is suspected in addition to stones in the bladder.

ii. A CBC, serum chemistry profile and urinalysis are indicated to rule out urinary tract infection and evaluate renal function.

An excretory urogram or ultrasound examination is performed to confirm ureteral stones are present.

iii. One option is to do serial radiographs and see if the ureteral calculus passes on its own. In a canine experimental study, solid spheres of 2.3 mm passed freely, 2.8 mm spheres became firmly impacted, and those of 3.9 mm or more could not even be introduced into the ureter. Given the size of the calculi here, the chances of it passing naturally are small.

If no irreversible damage is present in the kidney or ureter (e.g. marked hydronephrosis or hydroureter) a ureterotomy is performed to remove the calculus, and ventral cystotomy is performed to remove the bladder stones and flush the ureters. An intraoperative view of hydroureter with multiple calculi is shown (**14b**). Treatment with antibiotics (based on culture and sensitivity) and appropriate diet modification (based on calculi analysis) is indicated. After two weeks of ureteral obstruction an affected kidney will regain only 50–60% of its pre-obstruction function. With severe ureteral dilation, hydronephrosis or pyelonephritis, ureteronephrectomy is considered.

iv. Incise the ureter proximally because in most instances it is dilated and ureterotomy is easier; to close use simple interrupted or simple continuous sutures. Although gut, polyglycolic acid or polyglactin 9 have been used with success in the urinary tract, absorbable, 5-0 to 6-0, monofilament suture, such as polydioxanone (PDS, Ethicon) or polyglyconate (Maxon, Davis and Geck), with a swaged-on needle is recommended. These materials provide less tissue drag, better strength at a smaller size and varied pH, and induce less inflammation.

Stenting the ureters allows re-epithelialization if trauma has occurred. However, its use is controversial when good apposition is obtained. Any foreign body will increase local inflammation and ascending infection which both increase the risk of stenosis. The author (B. Bouvy) does not stent ureters routinely.

15 i. A seroma caused by: inadequate hemostasis or dead space closure; excessive tissue trauma from surgery or postoperative activity; or in this instance, failure to close the scapulohumeral joint capsule incision.

ii. Seromas delay wound healing by disruption of tissues; inhibition of reparative cells by local hypoxia, poor nutrient delivery and waste removal; and by serving as a medium for bacterial infection.

iii. Treatment options include open or closed drainage, pressure bandage support, and reduction of activity. Persistent lesions may require reoperation and surgical obliteration of dead space with sutures. Cytologic examination of the fluid is useful to rule out concurrent infection. The prognosis for recovery is good.

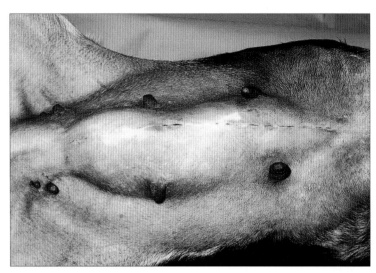

16a

16 This five-year-old, female, mixed-breed dog is presented three days after routine ovariohysterectomy (**16a**).
i. What is the presumptive diagnosis?
ii. What diagnostic tests could be performed to confirm the diagnosis?
iii. When is emergency surgery indicated?

17 A five-year-old Weimaraner (**17a**) presents with episodic weakness and is diagnosed as having persistent hypoglycemia (serum glucose <2.2 mmol/l (<40 mg/dl)). This patient exhibits 'Whipple's triad', and an insulin secreting tumor is suspected.
i. What is 'Whipple's triad'? Why are determinations of serum concentrations of both insulin and glucose helpful in ruling out other sources of hypoglycemia and diagnosing hyperinsulinemia?
ii. Describe surgery for an insulin secreting tumor.
iii. What medical alternatives are available for the treatment of islet cell tumors?

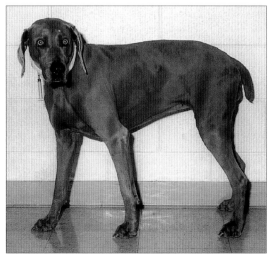

17a

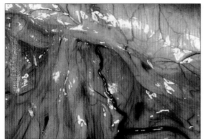

16 i. An abdominal wall dehiscence (16b).
ii. Digital palpation of the mass may reveal a hernia ring or allow the abdominal content to be reduced into the abdomen. Radiography and ultrasonography may prove valuable in confirming the diagnosis of incisional dehiscence and herniation of abdominal organs. Fine-needle aspiration biopsy helps rule out other soft tissue masses.
iii. Emergency surgery is indicated in cases that deteriorate despite medical supportive therapy, if the herniated organs show signs of obstruction or incarceration or when external wounds or fistulation are present.

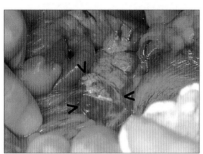

17 i. Whipple's triad consists of: symptoms after fasting or exercise; serum glucose concentration <2.8 mmol/l (50 mg/dl); symptoms relieved by the administration of glucose. Hypoglycemia may be caused by conditions other than an insulinoma (e.g. nonpancreatic neoplasms, pregnancy, hepatopathy, neonatal hypoglycemia). Hypoglycemia normally suppresses insulin secretion proportional to severity; islet cell tumors secrete insulin regardless of serum glucose concentrations. By finding concurrent low serum glucose and high insulin concentrations, one can determine whether or not hyperinsulinemia is present.
ii. The pancreas is carefully evaluated (17b) since islet cell tumors can be quite small (<0.5 cm). A detectable mass is excised by partial pancreatectomy. Metastatic disease is present at the time of surgery in as many as 45% of cases, and the liver is the most common site. The regional lymph nodes, liver and spleen are evaluated and excisional biopsy performed to evaluate for presence of metastatic disease and reduce tumour burden. If surgery is successful (complete excision of the islet cell tumor), then hypoglycemia should resolve. In one study 58% of patients became normoglycemic postoperatively and 27% remained hypoglycemic.
iii. Frequent feedings to maintain serum glucose levels and reduce exertional activity. Diazoxide inhibits insulin secretion, promotes hepatic gluconeogenesis resulting in increased glucose production, and stimulates the beta-adrenergic system reducing glucose utilization by antagonism at the cellular level. It is not cytotoxic to the neoplastic pancreatic islet cells and does not decrease insulin production. Streptozotocin selectively destroys pancreatic beta-cells and can be used for islet cell tumors but is potentially nephrotoxic. Glucocorticoids antagonize the effects of insulin at the cellular level and promote hepatic glycogenolysis resulting in increased serum glucose. Glucocorticoids are not cytotoxic but are useful in controlling the effects of hyperinsulinemia. Propranolol, a beta-adrenergic blocking agent, reduces insulin secretion by regulation of the beta-adrenergic nervous system. Unfortunately, it may also promote hypoglycemia by blocking hepatic gluconeogenesis.

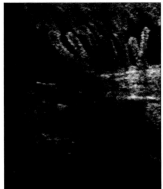

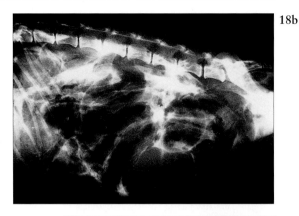

18 An abdominal sonogram (18a) of an 11-year-old, female, mixed-breed dog that presented with an abundant serosanguinous vulvar secretion of one month's duration. Onset was concomitant with late estrus. The sonogram shows cystic formations within a tubular structure. Polydipsia or polyuria was not present. A hemogram showed significant anemia and moderate leukocytosis (PCV 0.207 l/l (20.7%); Hb 63 g/l (6.3 g/dl); total protein 70 g/l (7.0 g/dl); RBCs 2.28 ×

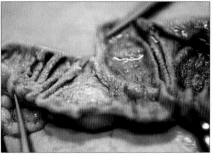

$10^{12}/l$ ($2.28 \times 10^6/mm^3$); leukocytes $29.4 \times 10^9/l$ ($29,400/mm^3$); neutrophils 91%). A lateral abdominal radiograph of the dog (18b) and the affected organ after surgical excision (18c) are shown.
i. What is the affected organ?
ii. What is your diagnosis?

19 A mandibular lesion was noted during oral examination of a ten-year-old, mixed-breed dog (19). The owner was concerned after seeing blood tinged saliva near the dog's water bowl.
i. What are the differential diagnoses for this lesion?
ii. What diagnostic tests would you perform?
iii. What treatment would you recommend?

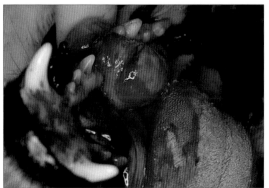

21

18 i. The fluid-filled structure in the caudal abdomen is the uterus. The presence of thin-walled cysts in the organ lumen is not a normal finding. When a contrast hysterogram is performed (18b), the uterus is visible as a dilated, fluid-filled mass occupying the caudal abdominal cavity. It is greatly distended and fluid in the lumen has diluted the contrast media (Iohexol – 300 mg I/ml). In the same image a small inguinal hernia is also evident. The radiographic image could be mistaken for a uterine perforation.

ii. Based on history, clinical signs, hemogram (neutrophylic leukocytosis and anemia from uterine hemorrhage) and radiograph and sonogram images, a diagnosis of cystic endometrial hyperplasia was made. Histologic evaluation of the uterus diagnosed Type II cystic endometrial hyperplasia. Type I hyperplasia is not associated with any particular phase of estrus and has minimal concurrent inflammatory response in the uterine wall. Type II hyperplasia is characterized by a uterine wall thickened from inflammatory cell infiltrates, cyst formation, occurrence during diestrus and a serosanguinous discharge (non-purulent). Type III hyperplasia is associated with marked inflammation (often purulent) and is the most common type associated with pyometra, and Type IV is chronic endometritis.

19 i. Squamous cell carcinoma, amelanotic melanoma, fibrosarcoma and epulis. Osteomyelitis is not usually associated with a mass lesion. Squamous cell carcinoma often appears as a flat, ulcerated, sessile lesion with a granular appearance such as this.

ii. The TNM system of tumor staging is used for animals with oral neoplasms. Tumor size and invasiveness based on clinical examination, regional radiographs, and sometimes computed tomography are used to determine the stage of the primary tumor (T). Incisional biopsy of oral tumors usually provides adequate tissue to determine the histologic diagnosis. For easily reached, protruding tumors on the labial sides of the mandible and maxilla a moderately deep wedge can be taken without anesthesia since tumors contain no nerves.

Regional lymph node metastases may occur in palpably normal lymph nodes. Regional nodes are assessed with a combination of palpation, fine-needle aspiration and cytology, and biopsy for histologic analysis (N). Lymph nodes with afferent drainage in this region are the mandibular, parotid and medial retropharyngeal nodes.

Ventrodorsal and right and left lateral thoracic radiographs of the chest are used to assess for the presence of thoracic metastases (M). A general health screen is also indicated to rule out concurrent disease which may affect prognosis or treatment strategy.

iii. Histologic diagnosis was squamous cell carcinoma, and staging showed the tumor was confined to the mandible (T2N0M0). Treatment options include surgical resection by rostral hemimandibulectomy, and radiation therapy. Local tumor control can be achieved in approximately 98% of cases and several reports claim total cure with a mean follow-up of 17 months after surgical excision. With radiation therapy, control rates of >50% at one year are reported. There is long-term risk of secondary malignancies after radiation therapy.

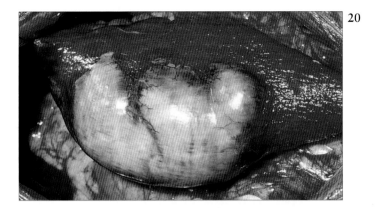

20

20 An exploratory laparotomy is performed on the dog in question 5. The stomach is repositioned, and the stomach wall is evaluated for viability.
i. The discoloration of the stomach wall (20) is often associated with what type of injury? Describe two possible surgical techniques to eliminate the problem.
ii. What clinical criteria are used to assess the presence and extent of ischemic injury to the stomach?
iii. The use of fluorescein dye to assess the gastric viability is controversial. What is the main reason for this controversy?

21 This open ulcerated lesion (21a) is present on the lateral aspect of the meta-tarsus in a six-year-old Great Dane. The lesion has been present for two years and has grown steadily over this period. The dog is not lame and the lesion is not irri-tating.
i. What is this lesion? What is the cause?
ii. How can it be treated? If surgery is necessary, describe the selected procedure.

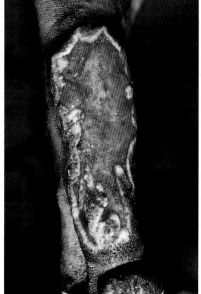

21a

20 i. Pale green to gray serosal areas are attributed to arterial or arteriovenous disruption and generally indicate ischemic or necrotic areas of the gastric wall that require surgical resection or partial gastric invagination.

ii. The criteria often used to evaluate the extent of gastric wall injury include serosal color and perfusion, gastric vascular patency and gastric wall texture. Active bleeding of the gastric wall after full thickness incision is used as the main criterion to determine the margin of resection.

iii. The use of fluorescein dye is not recommended because subserosal hemorrhage and corresponding serosal discoloration can block tissue fluorescence, resulting in a false-positive diagnosis of ischemic damage.

21b

21c

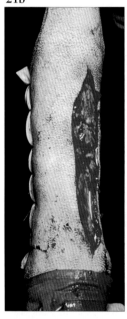 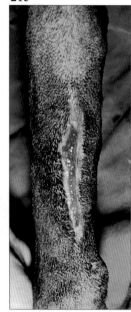

21 i. Pressure sores can develop over bony prominences in large breed dogs. The lesion typically progresses from skin edema and surface inflammation to a large raised ulcer from unsuccessful attempts of tissues to heal by contraction and epithelialization.

ii. With early pressure sores, the lesion is treated by protective bandage and soft bedding. If ulceration is limited, a callus will develop in many dogs. A large ulcer will not heal. Important considerations for correction are the limited amount of local skin and need for full thickness skin replacement because of continued pressure.

The simplest effective procedure is selected; a relaxing incision will allow closure of the large wound resulting from excision of the ulcer. An incision is made medially and extended until the surgeon determines that skin tension is not excessive (**21b**). This procedure has the additional advantage that the skin used to close the defect is from the local area and therefore resembles the original skin.

The relaxing incision, a bipedicle advancement flap, is used when the original defect must be closed with full thickness skin at the expense of an adjoining area. For this case the defect required strong, healthy skin and a scar on the medial aspect of the leg is not subjected to pressure. Most relaxing incisions heal well in animals by contraction and scarring is minimal. The relaxing incision is shown at day 25 (**21c**). Because of continued pressure on this area, recurrence of the ulcerated lesion is likely without continuous monitoring and treatment of the pressure sore before ulceration occurs.

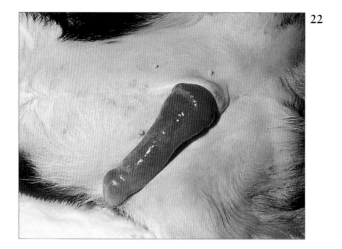

22

22 This dog (**22**) was presented for persistent erection. The penis cannot be reduced into the prepuce. No other physical abnormalities were found on examination.
i. What are the causes of this condition?
ii. What is the treatment for each of the above causes?

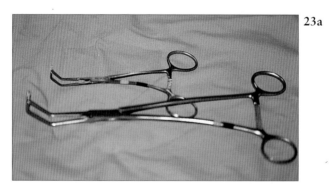

23a

23 Name this instrument (**23a**) and describe how it is used in vascular surgery.

24 Electrocautery is an extremely useful tool to the surgeon for rapid convenient hemostasis of small vessels. It provides a cleaner, blood-free field facilitating identi-fication of anatomic structures, and reduces blood loss from the patient (particularly important for very small animals). Describe how it works.

22 i. Paraphimosis, the inability to retract the erect penis following sexual stimulation, may be caused by an abnormally narrow preputial orifice (phimosis), a short prepuce, constriction by preputial hair, or trauma; strangulation resulting from placement of rubber bands or other constricting substance around the base of the erect penis; and priapism associated with local inflammation or, more commonly, spinal cord injury or disease.

ii. Paraphimosis is treated by cleaning and lubricating the penis and replacing it in the prepuce. Application of hyperosmolar solutions or warm packs are useful for shrinking the penis to facilitate replacement. For phimosis, surgical enlargement of the preputial orifice or partial penile amputation may be required to prevent recurrence.

Strangulation is treated by removing the strangulating object and treatment of the traumatized ischemic tissues. Catheterization may be needed to ensure urethral patency until resolution of penile edema.

The pathogenesis of priapism in man and dogs is not currently understood and treatment is limited. Treatment must be prompt and consists of preventing drying and self-trauma, and addressing the inciting cause (e.g. spinal fracture fixation). Injection of alpha-adrenergic drugs or benztropine, and anticholinergic drugs, into the corpus cavernosum penis to induce detumescence has been reported in man and a stallion. Surgical treatment in man is by creating a communication between the corpus cavernosum penis and the glans penis, and this may be an option in breeding animals.

Potential sequelae to chronic penile prolapse include penile necrosis and urethral obstruction. In these cases, partial or complete penile amputation is indicated.

23b

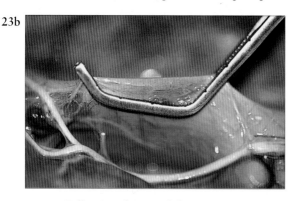

23 Satinsky vascular clamp. It is used to partially occlude atraumatically a blood vessel such as the vena cava allowing the surgeon to perform a lateral venotomy. The clamp is placed as demonstrated (**23b**) allowing blood to flow around the portion of the vein isolated by the clamp. The surgeon may then perform a venotomy for an end-to-side anastomosis or removal of an intraluminal mass such as a thrombus or tumor. Following closure of the venotomy or anastomosis, this atraumatic clamp is removed, thus re-establishing circulation.

24 Electrocautery works by passing high frequency alternating current through the body of the animal. The tissues provide resistance to current flow and a portion of the energy is converted to heat. Two electrodes of different sizes are used (the hand-piece and the ground plate) to concentrate current flow and provide greater energy density, and hence heat, at the smaller electrode. In bipolar cautery, both electrodes are in the hand piece and there is virtually no stray current allowing for more precise coagulation.

25 i. Identify this instrument (**25**).
ii. List common uses for this device.
iii. Are there alternative devices for some or all of these procedures?
iv. List the steps taken when using this instrument.

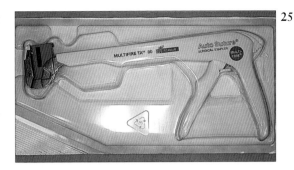

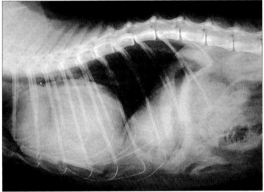

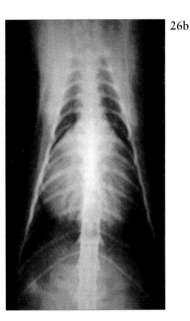

26 You are presented with a two-year-old, spayed female Cocker Spaniel with a history of lethargy and anorexia. Survey thoracic radiographs are shown (**26a, b**).
i. Describe the radiographic findings.
ii. What is the most likely diagnosis?
iii. How could you confirm this diagnosis?
iv. Describe the pathophysiology of this condition.
v. Describe the surgical treatment of this condition.
vi. What is the long-term prognosis following surgery for this patient?

25 i. Thoracoabdominal (TA) surgical stapler.

ii. Complete or partial lung lobectomy, atrial tumor resection, uterine stump ligation, partial hepatectomy, partial prostatectomy, enterotomy closure, gastrotomy closure and partial splenectomy are all common uses for this device.

iii. The gastrointestinal anastomosis (GIA) surgical stapler may be used for similar purposes. This stapler places a double row of staples and contains a blade to incise tissue between the staples.

iv. (1) Engage safety catch. (2) Open approximating lever. (3) Insert staple cartridge. (4) Stapler is placed over tissue to be stapled, approximating lever is closed. (5) Alignment is ensured, safety catch is disengaged and staple trigger is depressed. (6) Scalpel blade is used to excise tissue distal to the staple line and stapler is removed. (7) Staple line is inspected and additional sutures are placed as needed.

Some surgeons prefer to place a line of simple continuous suture over the line of staples for added security, especially when large vascular pedicles are present.

26c

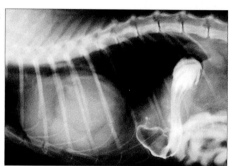

26 i. The cardiac silhouette is enlarged and contains opacities consistent with soft tissue and fat. The trachea is displaced dorsally. The liver shadow is not identified in the abdomen and loops of gas-filled intestine are in contact with the diaphragm. The diaphragm becomes indistinct ventrally.

ii. Peritoneopericardial diaphragmatic hernia.

iii. Echocardiography is best to confirm the diagnosis by imaging abdominal viscera such as spleen and liver within the pericardial sac. An upper gastrointestinal contrast radiographic study could also be used. In this case (**26c**) contrast approached the diaphragm but did not enter the pericardial sac; however, intestinal proximity to the diaphragm confirms the diagnosis, as normally the liver is interposed between these structures.

iv. Peritoneopericardial diaphragmatic hernia is usually congenital resulting from incomplete closure of the diaphragmatic septum transversum. Although present at birth, it often does not cause clinical signs until later in life and may be discovered incidentally. This defect is considered a developmental, not genetic or inherited, defect. Symptomatic patients generally have signs referable to the cardiopulmonary or gastrointestinal systems.

v. The hernia is accessed by ventral midline celiotomy. To reduce the hernia, the defect may need to be enlarged as the contents may be swollen. Adhesion of the hernia contents to the pericardium or epicardium is rare. Once reduced, the defect is closed using interrupted or continuous sutures with an absorbable material. Dorsal (deepest) sutures are placed first with closure continuing ventrally. Single layer closure is sufficient and it is not necessary to separate the pericardium from the peritoneum. Air is removed from the pericardial sac by aspiration through the suture line. This is especially important when the hernial sac is large and pneumopericardium could impair pulmonary expansion.

vi. Prognosis following herniorrhaphy is excellent.

27 i. Identify this instrument (27).
ii. What is its use?
iii. What precautions should be taken in using this instrument?

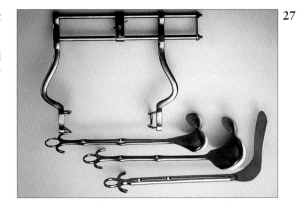

27

28 This is an oral view showing a chronic oronasal fistula in a dog (28a).
i. What are expected clinical signs associated with this lesion?
ii. How could this problem have been prevented?
iii. What are the surgical principles that maximize the incidence of a successful outcome?

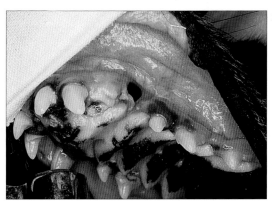

28a

29 The structures accessible through an intercostal thoracotomy vary with the intercostal space through which the approach is made. Identify the intercostal space and side of the chest most appropriate for an intercostal thoracotomy approach for surgical access to the following:
(a) Ductus arteriosus (patent ductus arteriosus or persistent right aortic arch).
(b) Caudal esophagus.
(c) Caudal vena cava.
(d) Feline thoracic duct.
(e) Canine thoracic duct.
(f) Cranial lung lobe.
(g) Intermediate lung lobe.
(h) Caudal lung lobe.
(i) Cranial esophagus.
(j) Pulmonic valve.

27 i. Balfour self-retaining abdominal retractor.
ii. Retraction of the abdominal wall to provide adequate visualization of the abdominal organs during surgery.
iii. The abdominal wall should be protected from drying and from blade trauma by using saline-soaked laparotomy sponges. Also, care must be taken to prevent entrapment of intestinal structures between the side blades and the abdominal wall.

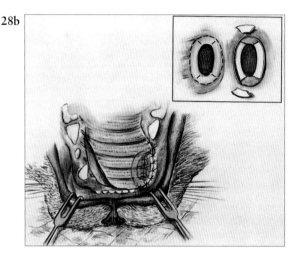

28b

28 i. Chronic rhinitis.
ii. Chronic oronasal fistula in this location is common secondary to extraction or spontaneous loss of the maxillary canine tooth. Minimal elevation of perialveolar mucogingival tissue and primary wound closure usually prevents oronasal fistula.
iii. A two layer closure is recommended for oronasal fistula repair. The first layer must provide an epithelial surface for the nasal cavity. This may be accomplished by elevating the periphery of the fistula and folding the oral epithelium inward. The second layer may be a buccal mucosa flap or a hard palate mucoperiosteal flap, providing the oral epithelial surface (**28b**) Other flap combinations may also be used successfully. Submucosal surfaces must be in apposition for healing; epithelium does not heal to epithelium.

29 (a) Left fourth intercostal space.
(b) Left or right 7–9th intercostal space.
(c) Right 7–9th intercostal space.
(d) Left 8–10th intercostal space.
(e) Right 8–10th intercostal space.
(f) Fifth intercostal space on the right or left side for the appropriate lung to be evaluated. In some cases, the 4th intercostal space may provide better access.
(g) Right 5th intercostal space. There is no intermediate lobe on the left side.
(h) Fifth intercostal space on the right or left side. In some cases, the 6th intercostal space may be used.
(i) Right 3rd or 4th intercostal space. The cranial esophagus cannot easily be accessed from the left side.
(j) Left 4th intercostal space.

30 A six-month-old, male Labrador Retriever puppy was brought to you for treatment of a closed femur fracture. The owner returns with the dog after ten days for suture removal. He comments that the dog has not been putting much weight on the leg. Vital signs are normal, with the exception of a body temperature of 40°C (104°F). On palpation, there is a fluid pocket present and the surgical incision appears red and inflamed. The dog resents palpation of the region.
i. What diagnostic tests would you use to confirm or deny the presence of a surgical wound infection?
ii. Describe in detail how you would perform those tests.
iii. What percentage of clean, closed fractures develop wound infection after surgery, and what organisms are most likely to be involved?
iv. What prophylactic antibiotic is recommended to decrease the incidence of infection in such a case?

31

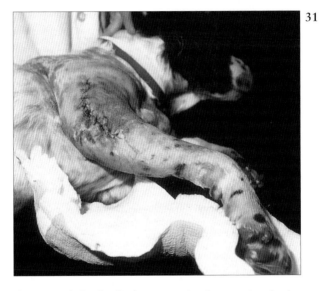

31 The lateral aspect of the forelimb one week after repair of a humeral condyle fracture (31).
i. Surgical apposition of tissues with sutures or staples immediately after wounding is classified as what type of wound closure or healing?
ii. This type of wound healing is characterized by what biological stages?

32 Patient hypothermia is a hazard that occurs during longer surgical procedures.
i. Which animals are at greatest risk?
ii. Describe several preventive measures.

30 i. The most useful test to confirm for infection at the surgical site is sterile aspiration of the fluid, cytologic examination and culture. A CBC might show evidence of inflammation, given that fever is present.

ii. In order to perform sterile aspiration, an area adjacent to the incision and outside the area of inflammation is clipped and surgically prepared. A sterile 22 gauge needle attached to a 6 ml syringe is directed through the surgically prepared skin into the fluid pocket. Fluid is withdrawn into the syringe and the needle withdrawn. The fluid sample is (1) placed into a vial containing transport media for bacterial culture, and (2) placed on glass slides for staining. The CBC is performed on blood drawn in a routine fashion.

iii. In a series of 1,399 clean fractures of the long bones and pelvis, an infection rate of 3.5% was documented. The organisms cultured most often from small animal surgical wounds are coagulase-positive staphylococci and *Escherichia coli*.

iv. Cefazolin (20 mg/kg given i/v at the start of surgery and s/c six hours later) is recommended for prophylaxis. This regime maintains the drug concentration at the surgical site above the MIC90 for coagulase-positive staphylococci and *Escherichia coli* for 12 hours.

31 i. Primary or first intention wound healing. With primary wound healing there is minimal wound contraction, epithelialization and scar formation. Also, because wound size is smaller, healing is more rapid. Second intention healing (or wound granulation) and third intention wound healing (delayed surgical closure of a granulating wound) are other forms of healing. They offer a potential advantage in infected wounds or where tissue is inadequate for primary closure, at the expense of greater scar tissue formation and longer healing time.

ii. Primary wound healing is characterized by the stages of inflammation (days 1–3), repair (days 4–14) and maturation (two weeks–many months). The inflammatory stage is characterized by neutrophil and macrophage influx to remove contaminants and cellular debris. Macrophages also produce essential cytokines that induce wound healing. The repair stage is characterized by capillary growth, fibroblast proliferation and collagen production. During the repair phase, wound strength is rapidly increasing. The maturation phase is characterized by remodelling of the scar, alignment of collagen fibers along lines of stress, and reduction in capillary density. The result is a more 'efficient' scar.

32 i. Small animals are at greater risk because of their relatively larger body surface area. Animals undergoing thoracic or abdominal surgery lose more heat because exposed viscera increase the surface area for radiation and evaporative heat loss, and critically sick animals often have subnormal temperatures before surgery requiring special measures to prevent further heat loss.

ii. Helpful measures include:

- Use of a heat pad (water blanket preferred).
- Warming intravenous fluids before administration or running the i/v line through hot water.
- Use of warm saline for body cavity lavage.
- Reducing surgical preparation time.
- Covering abdominal viscera with a sterile plastic bag to eliminate evaporation.
- Maintaining the animal on a closed or semi-closed anesthetic circuit to reduce ventilatory heat loss.

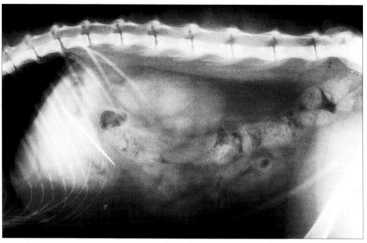

33a

33 A radiograph of the abdomen of a nine-month-old, domestic shorthair cat that has a history of severe vomiting for three days (**33a**).
i. The radiographic diagnosis is gastric foreign body. What laboratory tests would you perform, and what abnormal findings would you expect in a case like this?
ii. Describe the surgical technique for gastrotomy.
iii. What does the immediate after-care entail?

34 The larynx of a four-year-old, male Pug presented to the emergency clinic for dyspnea and cyanosis (**34**).
i. What is the diagnosis (be specific), and what is the cause of this problem?
ii. What other abnormalities may be present along with this condition in brachycephalic breeds?
iii. What treatment(s) are available, and what additional surgical procedures should be performed?

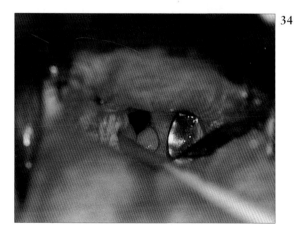

34

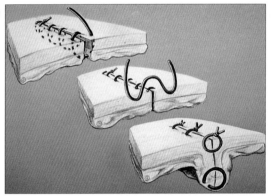

33b

33 i. Severe vomiting often leads to dehydration and electrolyte and acid-base disturbances. The most common abnormality is metabolic acidosis caused by fluid loss and decreased fluid intake. Routine laboratory evaluation should include measurement of hematocrit, electrolytes, acid-base status, BUN and creatinine.
ii. The gastrotomy incision is performed along a hypovascular region of the stomach, preferably on the ventral aspect of the gastric body midway between the greater and lesser curvatures. Stay sutures are placed at each end of the incision and the stomach is isolated with moist laparotomy sponges to contain spillage. The length of the incision depends on the size of the foreign body, for it must allow passage without tearing. Either a one-layer or a two-layer technique may be used to close the incision (**33b**). Use of synthetic, absorbable, monofilament material is preferred.
iii. Electrolyte solutions are administered intravenously to correct electrolyte and acid-base abnormalities. Water can be offered directly after surgery and feeding small amounts of food can be started as soon as 24 hours after surgery, if oral fluids are retained. The use of an antiemetic or of antimicrobial prophylaxis is usually not required.

34 i. Everted laryngeal saccules. This occurs secondary to chronic respiratory compromise of the upper airway. Increased respiratory effort from airway obstruction increases negative pressure at the glottis during inspiration, leading to eversion of the mucosa of the laryngeal saccules. This in turn exacerbates respiratory stridor.
ii. Brachycephalic airway syndrome is characterized by stenotic nares, elongated soft palate and everted laryngeal saccules arising from severe foreshortening of the skull in these breeds of dogs. Respiration can be further compromised by hypoplasia of the trachea. These primary factors may be accompanied chronically by secondary laryngeal collapse.
iii. Correction of everted laryngeal saccules is accomplished by grasping the everted saccule with a forcep (Babcock or Allis tissue) and surgically excising it with an instrument such as a tonsil snare, electroscalpel or scissors. Resection is simple and rapid, and improves breathing. Temporary tracheostomy can be performed to facilitate surgery and improve ventilation in the immediate postoperative period. Other surgical procedures performed concurrently include soft palate resection and correction of stenotic nares. If tonsilar enlargement and eversion has occurred, tonsillectomy is performed.

35 The inguinal area of a one-year-old, male Basset-hound is shown (35). The owner noted the mass only hours before when the dog was licking the area. The mass is soft and is associated with marked pain on palpation.
i. What are the differential diagnoses for this mass?
ii. What is the best treatment for this abnormality?

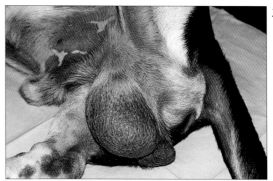

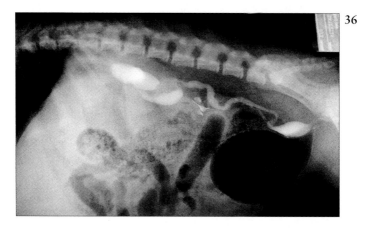

36 A 13-month-old, female English Bulldog is presented with a history of chronic recurrent urinary tract infection. In the past, clinical signs of pollakiuria and hematuria resolved when the dog was treated with antibiotics, but quickly recurred when therapy was stopped.
i. What diagnostic tests should be performed?
ii. An excretory urogram and negative contrast cystogram for this animal is shown (36). What is the diagnosis?
iii. What is the treatment for this abnormality?

37 i. Describe placement of a thoracostomy tube including the number of holes the tube should contain, the size of the tube, the location of the skin incision, the location of the thoracostomy, and the direction of insertion.
ii. What pressure should be used for aspiration through a thoracostomy tube?
iii. How much effusion does such a tube alone produce, and how does this influence a decision to remove the tube?

35–37: Answers

35 i. Differential diagnoses include testicular torsion, orchitis, testicular neoplasia and scrotal hernia. Definitive diagnosis is made by palpation, ultrasound examination and exploratory surgery. This dog has a scrotal hernia.
ii. Treatment for scrotal hernia involves reduction of hernial contents and imbrication of the vaginal process and inguinal ring; better still is to perform castration and complete closure of the vaginal process, and imbricate the inguinal ring allowing space only for the external pudendal vessels and genital nerve to pass. Recurrence of scrotal hernia is common if castration is not performed. The most common complications of herniorrhaphy and castration are scrotal dermatitis and hematoma formation.

36 i. Urine culture and sensitivity are performed to confirm infection and characterize antibiotic sensitivity. Unusual infections with mycoplasma or resistant bacterial strains must be considered, given the chronic recurrent history.

Imaging of the urinary tract is performed to rule out anatomic abnormalities, urinary calculi and prostatic disease in males where infections can be chronically harbored. Imaging choices include ultrasound examination and contrast radiography such as excretory urography and cystography. Ultrasound is generally more useful for kidney, bladder and prostate evaluation; contrast radiography is most helpful for ureteral, bladder and urethral abnormalities.
ii. The abnormality seen on the radiograph is a ureterocele. This is a cystic dilatation of the submucosal segment of the intravesicular ureter.
iii. Treatment for this abnormality is by surgical resection of the affected ureter and bladder wall, and reimplantation of normal, more proximal ureter into the bladder wall further cranial. If concurrent generalized hydroureter and advanced hydronephrosis is present, nephroureterectomy is performed.

37 i. The tube should be approximately the diameter of the mainstem bronchi and should contain at least five holes. The skin incision is made at the dorsal third of the 10th, 11th or 12th intercostal space. The tube is tunneled bluntly subcutaneously in a cranioventral direction to the level of the 7th or 8th intercostal space. The tube is introduced firmly in either the 7th or 8th intercostal space and fed into the cranioventral pleural space.
ii. The pressure used to aspirate through the tube should be between 10–20 cmH$_2$O. Excessive pressure can damage lung tissue.
iii. A few days after being placed, the presence of the tube alone will stimulate the production of 2–4 ml/kg/day of fluid. Red rubber tubes produce more than commercially available chest tubes. Once fluid production drops to this level, the clinician can assume that the fluid is a result of the tube and not the disease process. The tube can then safely be removed.

38 The external sheath of the rectus abdominus muscle of the dog shown (38) was closed with a simple continuous suture pattern. Compare the advantages and disadvantages of this method of closure with simple interrupted sutures.

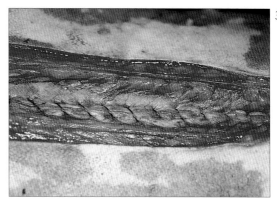

39 i. What is the diagnosis of the condition illustrated (39)?
ii. Where is the undescended testicle most likely located?
iii. What are four methods for retrieving an abdominally located testicle?
iv. List three reasons for removing cryptorchid testicles?

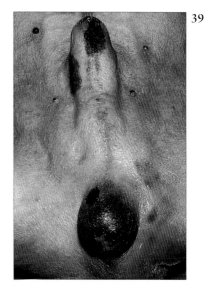

40 A six-year-old, female Boxer was presented for evaluation of a chronic draining tract on the left flank. The owners report a history of exposure to plant awns and the dog was normal when spayed at another hospital three weeks previously. On physical examination the dog's temperature was 39.6°C (103°F) and the abdominal wall tissues in the left flank were indurated and tender. Hemogram abnormalities included WBC, 27×10^9/l (27,000/mm³): 87% neutrophils, 5% lymphocytes and 8% monocytes.
i. What are the differential diagnoses for this lesion?
ii. What additional diagnostic test would be helpful?
iii. What is the treatment?

38 A simple interrupted suture pattern is classically used to close the external rectus sheath. Advantages of this technique include a safe, secure closure and correct apposition of the tissue borders. Disadvantages include time required for placement of the sutures, amount of suture material left in the wound and decreased suture economy. A simple continuous suture pattern has been more recently advocated for closure of the external rectus sheath because of adequate safety, decreased surgical time, decreased suture material left in the wound and increased suture economy. In one study evaluating simple continuous closure of the external sheath of the rectus abdominus muscle the incidence of dehiscence was 1/550 or 0.18%. Recommended sutures are monofilament polypropylene or polydioxanone, and sizes are 3-0 for patients under 2.5 kg, 2-0 for patients from 2.5–10 kg, and 0 for patients over 10 kg. Care is taken with either method of closure to include only the external rectus sheath as it is the holding layer of the abdominal wall, and inclusion of muscle in the suture line leads to necrosis and failure of the tissue to hold sutures.

39 i. Unilateral cryptorchidism.
ii. The most common location of a cryptorchid testicle is in the abdominal cavity. It can be located anywhere along the fetal tract of migration from a position near the cranial pole of the kidney to the external inguinal ring.
iii. The four methods are:

- The ductus deferens is traced from the prostatic termination to the testes.
- The testicular artery is traced from the aorta to the testicle.
- The testicular vein is traced from its termination on the caudal vena cava or left renal vein to the testicle.
- The gubernaculum testes is retrieved with a Snook hook, in the same manner as retrieving a uterine horn, and traced to the testicle.

iv. The three reasons are:

- Intact cryptorchid males are 13.6 times more likely to develop testicular tumors (Sertoli cell tumors, seminomas) than non-cryptorchid males.
- Cryptorchid males are more likely to develop testicular torsion.
- The trait is heritable.

40 i. A fistulous tract – foreign body reaction due to either a plant awn such as a foxtail that has migrated into the body wall, or use of braided non-absorbable suture (e.g. caprolactam) to ligate the ovarian pedicles during ovariohysterectomy.
ii. A contrast fistulogram can aid identification of the size, location and source of origin of the fistulous tract. Occasionally, a foreign body can be seen as a filling defect in the contrast shadow. Ultrasound is also reportedly useful for identification of fistulous tracts and detection of foreign objects.
iii. Treatment of fistulous tracts can be difficult and frustrating. If the source of the lesion is identified and removed by surgical exploration, routine drainage and wound management will resolve the clinical signs. For a fistulous tract arising from ovariohysterectomy, exploratory laparotomy is performed and the inciting ligature removed. If the source of a tract cannot be identified, en bloc removal of all affected tissues is indicated; recurrent tracts are common and owners must be advised that multiple surgeries may be required when the primary cause is not definitively identified.

41 You are planning to perform a cystotomy on a six-year-old, castrated male domestic shorthair cat.
i. What preoperative/operative pain control drugs will you choose?
ii. How will you monitor for postoperative pain?
iii. What postoperative pain control therapy will you provide?

42 You are presented with a seven-year-old English Springer Spaniel with a history of exercise intolerance and 'passing out'. On physical examination the dog is alert and active. On auscultation of the heart you determine that there is bradycardia (heart rate 55 bpm). The lead II electrocardiogram (ECG) you recorded for this patient is shown (**42**).
i. Name the arrhythmia and describe its features.
ii. What are the potential causes of this arrhythmia?

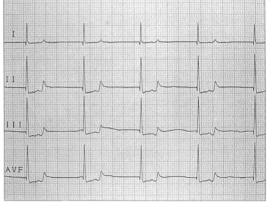

iii. If this dogs electrolytes are normal, how would you treat it?

43 A mass on the flank of an eight-year-old mixed-breed dog is shown (**43**). The owners first noted the mass one month previously and it has grown approximately 25% in size since that time. The dog has no clinical signs related to the mass.
i. What are the differential diagnoses, and what procedure will establish the definitive diagnosis?
ii. If this mass was diagnosed as a hemangiopericytoma what treatments could be considered, and what are the risks and benefits of each?
iii. If surgery was chosen for treatment, describe specifically how you would manage the case.

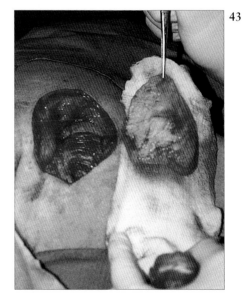

41–43: Answers

41 i. Oxymorphone (0.05 mg/kg i/v, i/m or s/c), butorphanol (0.4 mg/kg i/v, i/m or s/c) and xylazine (1 mg/kg i/m) all provide some degree of analgesia. The first two drugs would be more appropriate for a cat undergoing a major abdominal surgery, since there are fewer cardiovascular side-effects.
ii. Cats are difficult to monitor because their behavioral response to pain is that of a solitary animal: they lie still and dissociate from their environment. If provoked by palpation or manipulation, they may vocalize or become vicious. Ideally, the cat should remain calm, be able to sleep comfortably and display normal greeting behavior after ovariohysterectomy. High heart rates after surgery may be due to pain, but can also be from other stresses (hospitalization, cardiovascular instability).
iii. Oxymorphone (0.05 mg/kg i/v, i/m or s/c, q 3–4 hours) can be used. If narcotic-induced delirium occurs, administer acepromazine (0.025–0.05 mg/kg i/v, i/m or s/c, q 3–4 hours). Butorphanol (0.4 mg/kg i/v, i/m or s/c, q 1–2 hours) may be used, but the sedative effects often last 3–4 hours, which confounds patient monitoring.

42 i. This ECG is consistent with atrial standstill. The features of atrial standstill are bradycardia (usually less than 60 bpm), absence of P waves in all leads and normal appearing QRS complexes initiated from a supraventricular focus.
ii. Hyperkalemia associated with Addison's disease, oliguric renal failure and obstructive uropathy can cause atrial standstill. Other rule outs include digitalis toxicity and persistent atrial standstill. Persistent atrial standstill occurs most commonly in English Springer Spaniels. Its etiology remains undetermined; however, an underlying muscular dystrophy has been described in some dogs with persistent atrial standstill. These dogs demonstrate atrial standstill on ECG, but have normal electrolytes and the rate does not increase after the administration of atropine.
iii. The treatment of choice is permanent ventricular pacemaker implantation.

43 i. Differential diagnoses include neoplasia, abscess, granuloma, hematoma/seroma and abdominal hernia. Specific neoplasms to consider include soft tissue sarcoma, mast cell tumor, fibroma and lipoma. Definitive diagnosis is reached by a combination of palpation, fine-needle aspirate, and biopsy if a solid mass is identified and fine-needle aspirate was not helpful.
ii. Treatment options for hemangiopericytoma include wide surgical resection (local control 85–90%) and radiation with or without adjuvant hyperthermia. Because metastatic rates for hemangiopericytoma are less than 10%, treatment with systemic chemotherapy is not warranted. Local tumor control rates are approximately 50% with radiation. The main risk of surgery is incomplete resection; for radiation it is the poorer response rates and occurrence of secondary malignancies (<10%).
iii. Surgical resection of a soft tissue sarcoma requires wide or radical margins. These tumors are prone to extensive local invasion. Tumors are removed completely contained within an envelope of normal tissue. Collagen-rich, vascular-poor tissues (e.g. fascia, cartilage etc.) are utilized as biologic barriers to ensure complete tumor-free lateral and deep margins. The surgical wound is closed primarily or, if the wound is large, with a combination of polypropylene mesh, muscle flap and axial pattern skin flap as needed to ensure a tension-free closure.

44 A tumor located in the greater curvature of the stomach of a dog is shown (**44**).
i. What is the most common type of stomach tumor found in dogs?
ii. What other types of tumors are included in your differential diagnoses?
iii. What is the prognosis for this dog after complete excision of the tumor?

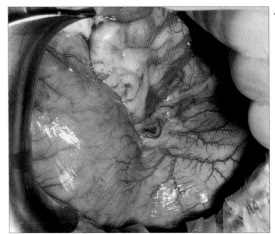

45 A six-year-old, castrated male Golden Retriever was presented with a four week history of progressive stranguria. A partial obstruction was appreciated on catheterization of the urethra. A urethrogram confirmed a well circumscribed mass in the prescrotal urethra.
i. What is the surgical procedure shown (**45**)?
ii. Describe a surgical treatment for this mass if the lesion was benign, and another if it was malignant.
iii. Describe any special postoperative requirements for these surgical procedures.

46 When selecting sutures for different tissue types, what are the preferred types and sizes:
i. For skin?
ii. For subcutis?
iii. For fascia?

44 i. Gastric adenocarcinoma (comprises 42–72% of stomach tumors in dogs).
ii. Leiomyosarcoma, lymphoma, fibrosarcoma, leiomyoma and adenoma. Diagnosis is made by endoscopic or surgical biopsy.
iii. The prognosis is poor when there is invasion to the serosal surface. Metastatic sites include regional lymph nodes (50–70%), liver (10–30%) and other sites such as lungs, omentum and peritoneum (<20%). Early stage disease can be cured, while treatment of late stage disease results in survival time of 5–12 months. Early detection, accurate staging and complete en bloc resection of all tumor is important to providing the best outcome.

45 i. A prescrotal urethrotomy.
ii. If the mass was benign, as in this case, excision or permanent urethrostomy proximal to the site of obstruction is considered. If the lesion was malignant, then segmental urethral excision or penile amputation is recommended.

In dogs, urethrostomy can be performed in the penile (prescrotal), scrotal, perineal or antepubic urethra. Urinary scalding is common after perineal urethrostomy in dogs and is probably best avoided.

When performing urethral incision or resection, meticulous technique is important to prevent stricture and minimize hemorrhage. Urethral epithelium is carefully apposed (whether to itself for urethrotomy, or to the skin for urethrostomy) with 4-0 or 5-0 monofilament suture in a simple interrupted pattern. Castration is performed on intact animals undergoing permanent urethrostomy to prevent erection.
iii. After urethrostomy the most common complication is hemorrhage or self trauma. An Elizabethan collar is used until the time of suture removal. Hemorrhage is minimized by using cold packs and sedation to minimize excitement. The surgical site is not cleaned and no attempts are made to remove blood clots or crusts.

After urethrotomy or segmental resection, stricture and dehiscence are the most common complications. A soft indwelling urinary catheter can be placed for 7–10 days to provide urinary bypass and stenting if the surgeon is concerned. If the urethral tissues are healthy and epithelial apposition is good, then no catheter is needed. If there is detrusor atony, bethanecol (5–30 mg p/o q 8 hours) is administered.

46 i. Monofilament nylon and polypropylene are the preferred sutures for skin. Braided materials or sutures that are reactive should be avoided. In selecting suture size, one should choose the smallest size suture possible that has strength comparable to the tissue being sutured. Use of too large a suture results in excessive foreign material in the wound and needlessly alters the architecture of the sutured tissue. 3-0 or 4-0 is the appropriate size for skin in small animal surgery.
ii. Monofilament absorbable sutures are preferable for subcutis. 3-0 or 4-0 is the appropriate size.
iii. Monofilament nylon and polypropylene, as well as surgical gut and synthetic absorbable sutures, have also been used effectively in fascia, although the latter two materials do not have prolonged suture strength. Appropriate sizes for small animals range from 0 to 3-0.

47

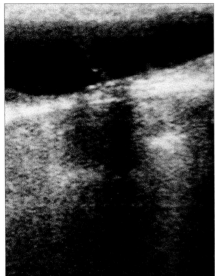

48

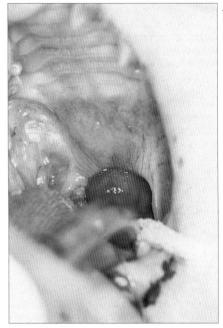

47 A seven-year-old, female, mixed-breed dog is presented with a distended abdomen, polydipsia/polyuria and progressive anorexia and lethargy. At this time there is no vulvar secretion but the owners recall the dog having a thick yellowish discharge 10–12 days previously that quickly disappeared. Last estrus was ten weeks ago. A caudal abdominal sonogram is shown (47).
i. What is the suspected diagnosis?
ii. What other procedures would you consider to confirm the diagnosis?
iii. What is the treatment of choice?

48 A mass in the naso- and oropharyngeal region in a 11-month-old cat is shown (48).
i. What would be the predominant clinical sign?
ii. What is the diagnosis and why is it often misdiagnosed?
iii. What diagnostic tests should be performed to determine the extent of the lesion?

49 A five-year-old, male domestic shorthair cat is presented for urinary obstruction. It is the fourth episode in six months. The owners report difficulty complying with dietary and medical recommendations previously prescribed for feline urolithiasis syndrome (FUS), and are becoming frustrated by their frequent trips to the veterinarian to treat the obstructions.
i. What surgical treatment is available?
ii. Briefly describe the procedure.
iii. What are the potential complications?

47 i. Closed pyometra. The history of purulent vaginal discharge and the time since last estrus strongly support the diagnosis. Pyometra generally occurs between 9–12 weeks after estrus when the uterus is under progesterone influence from an active corpus luteum. The sonogram shows a dilated, fluid-filled uterus typical of pyometra.
ii. The sonogram in this case is sufficient for diagnosis. A hemogram, serum chemistry profile and urinalysis would help support the diagnosis (presence of a neutrophilia and mild anemia) and allow evaluation of hydration status, electrolyte balance and renal and hepatic function. Up to 50% of animals have concurrent nephropathy or hepatopathy, and most dogs have concurrent bacterial cystitis.
iii. Ovariohysterectomy. Use of antibiotics and prostaglandins (PGF2) is not advised in this case because of the extensive uterine dilation and closed cervix. This treatment can cause peritonitis from uterine rupture or reflux of purulent material up the uterine horns. Medical management is appropriate only for open pyometra when an owner declines ovariohysterectomy because they desire to breed the bitch.

48 i. Chronic rhinitis.
ii. Nasopharyngeal polyp. The common misdiagnosis is viral upper respiratory infection. Usually viral infections resolve with time and appropriate supportive care. When symptomatic therapy is discontinued in patients with a nasopharyngeal polyp, the clinical signs recur.
iii. Nasopharyngeal polyps originate in the dorsomedial compartment of the tympanic bulla. The lesion may extend down the Eustachian tube to enter the nasopharynx or up the external ear canal. Otoscopic examination and bulla radiographic series aid in assessing the invasiveness of the polyp. The pharyngeal and aural components may be avulsed manually and removed. However, if there is radiographic evidence of a soft tissue mass in the bulla, exploratory ventral bulla osteotomy is indicated. Surgery for nasopharyngeal polyp may be associated with transient ipsilateral Horner's syndrome.

49 i. Perineal urethrostomy. Owners should be advised that perineal urethrostomy will prevent urinary obstruction but will not resolve signs of FUS, and that adjunct medical management will still be required.
ii. An elliptical incision is made around the prepuce and scrotum and the penis is dissected free from the subcutaneous tissues. The ischiocavernosus muscles are transected and the pelvic ligaments bluntly dissected to free the penis to the level of the bulbourethral glands where the urethral diameter is significantly larger. The retractor penis muscle is reflected and the urethra is incised dorsally. The urethral mucosa is meticulously apposed to the skin with small (4-0 or 5-0) interrupted nonabsorbable sutures, creating a new, larger stoma that will allow the passage of urethral plugs and small stones. The penis is amputated distally leaving a short 'drain board' of urethral mucosa ventral to the orifice. An Elizabethan collar is placed until the time of suture removal.
iii. Reported complications are persistent hemorrhage, dehiscence, self-mutilation, cystitis and urethral stricture if the urethra is not opened at the level of the bulbourethral glands or if the skin and urethral mucosa are not meticulously apposed. If the cat has been chronically obstructed, preoperative diuresis for management of azotemia may be required to minimize anesthetic risk.

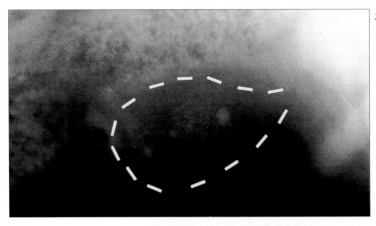

50a

50 A 12-year-old, castrated male Keeshound with recurrent urinary tract infections is identified as having cystic calculi (50a). Cystotomy was performed and calculi analysis identified the stones as calcium oxalate (50b). A preoperative serum chemistry profile revealed hypercalcemia.

i. What are the most common pathologic conditions that result in hypercalcemia?
ii. Describe a systematic approach to determining the cause of hypercalcemia?

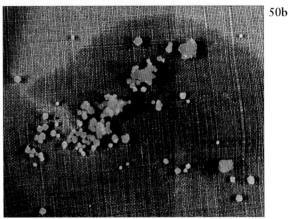

50b

51 You are presented with a four-year-old, female domestic shorthair cat that is anorexic, depressed and febrile. She has vomited occasionally over the last week. On palpation of the abdomen you feel the intestines bunched and crowded into the cranial abdomen. You examine the base of the tongue and can see what appears to be a thin ridge of granulation tissue on the ventral aspect (see also 194).
i. What condition is being described and what is the most likely reason for the depression, anorexia and fever? How would you confirm or deny your suspicions?
ii. What contaminating organisms are likely to be associated with this condition?
iii. What antibiotic therapy is instituted before surgical correction of the problem?

50 i. Renal failure (acute and chronic); humoral hypercalcemia of malignancy (e.g. lymphoma, anal sac apocrine gland adenocarcinoma); hypoadrenocorticism; osteolytic conditions (e.g. neoplastic, osteomyelitis); hypervitaminosis D; primary hyperparathyroidism (parathyroid adenoma, hyperplasia).
ii. History is used to rule out vitamin toxicoses, dietary imbalances, or rodenticide ingestion inducing hypervitaminosis D. Physical examination is performed to identify any neoplasia (e.g. lymphadenopathy, painful bone lesions, anal gland tumors, etc.). Clinicopathologic testing includes a CBC, serum chemistry profile and urinalysis. A CBC is helpful to diagnose lymphoma or leukemia. The serum chemistry profile and urinalysis are evaluated for signs of renal failure, hepatopathy, electrolyte imbalance (hypoadrenocorticism) or hyperglobulinemia and proteinuria (multiple myeloma). Further evaluation for multiple myeloma includes protein electrophoresis, bone marrow evaluation and survey radiography to check for lytic bone lesions can be pursued. Hypoadrenocorticism is confirmed by performing an ACTH stimulation test.

Thoracic and abdominal imaging help to identify internal lymphadenopathy or skeletal changes inducing hypercalcemia of malignancy. If all tests are normal, primary hyperparathyroidism is considered and a parathyroid hormone assay is performed. Surgical exploration of the parathyroid glands can be both diagnostic and therapeutic.

51

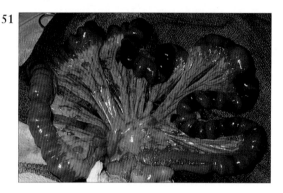

51 i. Peritonitis secondary to linear foreign body. The ridge of granulation tissue at the base of the tongue is associated with a string cutting deeply into the tissues. The bunching of the intestines is due to plication over the string (**51**). Peritonitis occurs when the string, which embeds into the mesenteric side of the intestine, cuts or erodes through the intestinal wall. Vomiting is due to both obstruction and peritoneal irritation, while anorexia and fever are most likely associated with peritonitis. Prognostic tests of value include CBC, survey abdominal radiographs to look for signs of plication, and contrast (iodine or barium) enterogram if survey radiograph results are equivocal. If perforation is suspected, abdominocentesis or abdominal lavage is performed to recover a sample for cytologic analysis.
ii. A mixture of organisms including anaerobes such as *Bacteroides*, *Clostidium* and *Fusobacterium* and Gram-negative enteric organisms and enterococci are usually present. Bacterial concentrations are normally 5–6 log values higher in the lower gastrointestinal tract than in the upper tract, although this ratio narrows under conditions of obstruction.
iii. Cefoxitin (30 mg/kg, i/v, q 5 hours, given slowly to avoid vomiting) or cefotetan (30 mg/kg, i/v, q 8 hours) have activity against anaerobes and Gram-negative enteric bacteria, but less activity against enterococci. Combinations of an aminoglycoside (gentamicin, amikacin), plus an anti-anaerobe drug (clindamycin, metronidazole), plus or minus ampicillin (which has activity against enterococci) can also be used.

52 What is the advantage of initiating early enteral feeding in animals after surgery?

53 This is a postoperative oral view of a surgery site for cleft hard palate repair in a dog (53).
i. What is the name and basis for the surgical procedure performed?
ii. Will lateral oronasal defects secondary to medial movement of palate muco-periosteum heal without further surgery?
iii. What is the prognosis for this disease?

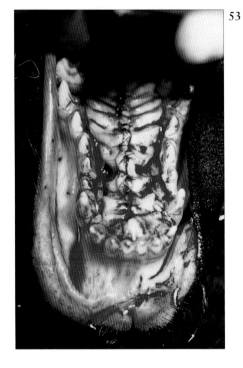

53

54 You are presented with a five-year-old, spayed female Shetland Sheepdog which has just been hit by a car. During your physical examination, crackles within the lung fields are heard on auscultation. Additionally, you notice that a section of the chest wall in the same area seems to move in during inspiration and out during expiration.
i. What is your tentative diagnosis based on this paradoxical respiratory movement, and what is the mechanism for this paradoxical motion?
ii. How should this condition be managed?

52 The advantage of feeding soon after surgery (even for animals undergoing gastrointestinal tract surgery) is that it promotes metabolic anabolism and a healthy intestinal mucosa. It is important to prevent systemic catabolism because calories and amino acids in an unfed animal are soon derived from endogenous sources. Since there are no natural protein stores in the body, functional resources (e.g. immune and visceral proteins) are used, resulting in reduced immune defense, metabolism and wound healing. In humans, nutritional support is documented to reduce postoperative morbidity and mortality for many procedures. Enteral feeding is important to enterocyte nutrition, promotion of healthy intestinal mucosa, and reduced bacterial translocation from the gut (an important source of postoperative sepsis). Enterocytes receive 40–70% of their nutrition from the gut lumen and the balance from the systemic blood supply. Colonocytes preferentially use short chain fatty acids and small intestinal enterocytes use glutamine obtained from the lumen for sustenance.

53 i. The surgery performed in this dog was a modified Van Langenbeck technique. The surgical basis for this technique is the development of lateral relief incisions to prevent tension on the sutured defect. The defect is sutured in two layers (see **190**).
ii. Lateral oronasal defects may be present postoperatively, especially in dogs with wide defects of the maxillary bones. These defects generally heal spontaneously without the need for further surgery.
iii. The prognosis for surgical closure of cleft hard palate is good, however owners should be made aware that multiple procedures may be required to attain complete defect closure.

54

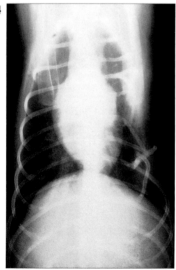

54 i. Flail chest. This occurs when multiple rib fractures result in a free unsupported section of thoracic wall (**54**). When the patient inhales, the chest expands and as negative intrapleural pressure is generated the free section is pulled inward, opposite to the direction of the remainder of the chest. When the patient exhales the chest collapses generating a positive intrapleural pressure, and the free segment is forced outward while the remainder of the chest collapses.
ii. In most cases, flail chest is associated with severe chest trauma and the patient should be stabilized prior to treatment. Hypoxemia is often secondary to ventilation/perfusion mismatch and the presence of pulmonary contusion. An external splint may be used for temporary or definitive treatment of flail chest. An aluminum bar splint is fashioned to fit around the neck and along the sides of the chest connected over the lumbar spine. A suture is placed blindly around the ribs of the free section and secured to the splint. If this treatment is to be the definitive treatment, the splint should be left in place for 4–6 weeks to allow the ribs to heal. Alternatively, the ribs may be approached surgically, reduced and stabilized primarily.

55 The testicles of a ten-year-old dog that presented for testicular enlargement are shown (55). The testicle was firm and non-painful on examination. The remainder of the physical examination was normal.
i. What are the differential diagnoses?
ii. What additional diagnostic tests or staging procedures are indicated?
iii. What is the prognosis?

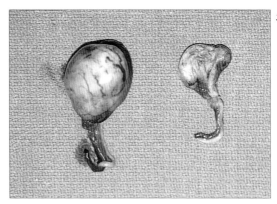

56 A nine-year-old, male Miniature Poodle presents with intermittent hematuria, foul smelling urine and lumbar pain. The dog's appetite is poor. Although you suspect cystic or urethral calculi, urethral catheterization and contrast cystourethrography appear normal.
i. Are urinary calculi definitely ruled out? If not, what type of calculi is suspected?
ii. Upon more careful scrutiny of abdominal radiographs you suspect radiopaque structures are present in the kidneys. Is this diagnostic? Which tests are now indicated?
iii. Having diagnosed bilateral nephroliths, moderate renal failure and pyelonephritis, should you treat this animal medically or surgically?

57 A four-year-old, castrated male domestic shorthair cat that presented for this ulcerative lesion on the upper lip is shown (57). The lesion is non-painful and non-pruritic. What is the diagnosis and list one differential that should be considered?

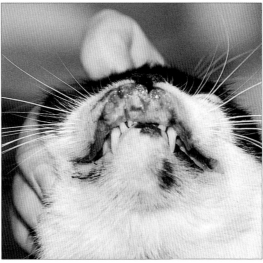

55 i. Sertoli cell tumor, seminoma and interstitial cell tumors are the most common testicular tumors, although fibrosarcoma, granulosa cell tumor, hemangiosarcoma, leiomyoma, schwannoma, undifferentiated sarcoma/carcinoma and gonadoblastoma have been reported. Other causes of testicular enlargement (e.g. torsion, orchitis, scrotal hernia) are excluded because the testes are not painful on palpation.
ii. A CBC is performed since testicular tumors, especially sertoli cell tumors, can produce estrogens and may cause blood dyscrasias such as anemia, thrombocytopenia and pancytopenia. Metastasis of the most common testicular tumors is rare (9% Sertoli cell tumors, 4% seminomas and 0.6% interstitial cell tumors) and usually affects the sublumbar and inguinal lymph nodes. Staging includes at least palpation and perhaps ultrasound examination of these nodes. Fine-needle or other type biopsy is performed if lymphadenopathy is detected.
iii. Sertoli cell tumors, seminomas and interstitial cell tumors without blood dyscrasias or lymph node involvement warrant a good prognosis following castration. Blood dyscrasias worsen the prognosis because they may persist for months after the tumor is removed. Radiation therapy for lymph node metastasis has been successful for these tumors.

56 i. Although uncommon (1.3–4% of canine urinary calculi), uroliths can be in the renal pelves (2.5% bilaterally) or ureters. When present in the upper urinary tract, concurrent calculi of the lower urinary tract occur in 47% of male and 23% of female dogs. Nephroliths are most commonly composed of calcium salts (65% oxalate and phosphate) and often have no associated clinical signs.
ii. Other radiopaque structures may resemble nephroliths on abdominal radiographs (e.g. intestinal content, calcified lymph node, mineralization of renal diverticula), and stones with low calcium content are radiolucent (e.g. urates, silicates). Abdominal ultrasonography is used to confirm nephrolithiasis and rule out secondary hydronephrosis or concurrent pyelonephritis. Excretory urography is an alternative if ultrasonography is not available. It requires uncompromised renal blood flow and function to excrete iodine contrast in enough concentration to produce a good quality study. Urinalysis, hemogram, and serum chemistry profile are indicated to evaluate renal function and test for urinary tract infection. Other useful tests include urine culture and urine protein quantitation.
iii. Detection of nephroliths alone is not a direct indication for surgery. Removal is indicated when there is refractory infection, obstruction of the renal pelvis, progressive enlargement or failed attempts at medical/dietary dissolution of stones, or deterioration of renal function. Other special circumstances where surgery may be indicated are in growing animals because the safety of low-protein/low-magnesium diets is not proven, and in males where acute urethral obstruction is a risk.

57 i. Feline eosinophilic granuloma complex (EGC) – eosinophilic or rodent ulcer. This lesion should not be confused with eosinophilic plaques which are most commonly found over the abdomen and groin, or linear granulomas (eosinophilic collagenolytic granulomas) which are most common in young cats and are found over the caudal thighs and in a nodular form in the oral cavity. Linear granulomas also occur on the nose, chin, lips, pinnae, foot pads or paws. Important differential diagnoses to consider are oral squamous cell carcinoma, plasma cell stomatitis-pharyngitis and oral gingivitis, periodontitis and stomatitis from viral infections.

58 With regard to the cat in question **57**:
i. What test(s) will be most useful in confirming the diagnosis?
ii. List three treatments that are available for management of this syndrome?

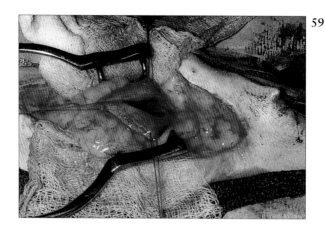

59

59 The dog illustrated (**59**) had a cystotomy for removal of a struvite urolith that was present for six months.
i. What suture material is appropriate for closure of this cystotomy?
ii. What suture materials are inappropriate for closure of this cystotomy?
iii. What suture patterns are acceptable for closing this cystotomy?

60 An intraoperative photograph is shown of a five-year-old, female Schnauzer with a two month history of coughing and weight loss that has been non-responsive to antibiotic therapy (**60**). A tentative diagnosis of pulmonary abscess has been made.
i. What is the surgical course of action?
ii. Are there any concerns with this?
iii. What is the prognosis?

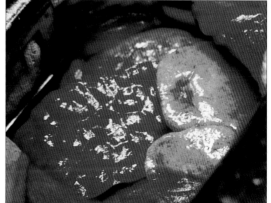

60

58 i. Tissue biopsy, hemogram (peripheral eosinophilia is most commonly seen with eosinophilic plaques and linear granulomas), serum titers for FeLV and FIV virus, and elimination diet to rule out food allergy as the cause. Histopathologic analysis will identify specific tissue patterns to differentiate each of the subclinical divisions of EGC, and will rule out neoplasia and plasma cell stomatitis-pharyngitis.
ii. Corticosteroid therapy: methylprednisolone acetate (i/m) or prednisone (p/o). Antihistamine therapy: chlorpheniramine and hydroxyzine hydrochloride are most commonly used when atopy and flea allergy are considered contributory. Food antigen management: is implemented after determining a dietary source of allergy. Hyposensitization has little efficacy in the cat but some cases of EGC due to feline atopy may respond. Antibiotic therapy is used to treat secondary pyoderma. Antibiotics commonly used include trimethoprim-sulfa, amoxicillin-clavulinate and cephalosporins. Progesterone compounds are not recommended because of associated side effects.

59 i. Absorbable sutures are used whenever possible in the urinary bladder to reduce risk of adhesions, infection and urolith production. Struvite urolithiasis is indicative of a bacterial infection; in one *in vitro* report evaluating suture strength in infected urine, polydioxanone retained greatest breaking strength.
ii. The above study showed that no suture material retains excellent breaking strength. Polyglactin 910, polyglycolic acid and chromic gut did not retain sufficient strength to allow healing in urine infected with *Proteus* spp. Braided suture material can act as a wick for infection and is inappropriate for this case. Non-absorbable suture is also inappropriate (see i. above).
iii. The suture pattern selected for closure of the urinary bladder should be watertight, technically simple to perform, provide anatomic reconstruction, avoid penetrating the mucosa, and not cause significant decrease in lumen size. Simple interrupted closure incorporating the submucosa in one layer and seromuscular layers in another, accomplishes these goals. This suture pattern has similar bursting wall strength to double layer inverting patterns, but with more anatomic alignment of tissues and less decrease in lumen diameter. Double layer inverting closure is probably better suited to closure of defects when the healing capacity of the bladder is questionable. A single layer appositional closure is adequate for a healthy bladder.

60 i. Complete pulmonary lobectomy of the abscessed lobe is performed. The lung lobe or lobes are submitted for histopathologic and microbiologic analysis to define the etiologic agent. Surgical stapling devices are ideal for performing lobectomy as they minimize operative time and manipulation of the affected lung. Extensive manipulation of the abscessed lung can cause drainage of purulent material into adjacent unaffected lobes, and potentially cause occlusion of major airways and life-threatening complications.
ii. Every effort is made to manage this condition via antimicrobials and supportive therapy. A mortality rate of 20.3% was noted in one study, and dogs treated medically for more than 1.3 months prior to surgery had a significantly greater survival rate. Also, a significant increase in mortality was noted with increasing number of pulmonary lobes removed. Interestingly, the etiologic agent isolated did not have a significant effect on the final outcome.
iii. The prognosis is fairly good for animals surviving the perioperative period: approximately 25% mortality rate, 50% have complete resolution with surgery, and 25% unresolved or recurrent pneumonia.

61 An 18-year-old, spayed female cat is presented for bilateral thyroidectomy. The cat has been managed medically with methimazole therapy; however, the side-effects have become intolerable. On examination, heart rate is 150 bpm, respirations are normal and the cat is well hydrated. The following preoperative laboratory results are obtained: PCV 0.36 l/l (36%); serum protein 62 g/l (6.2 g/dl); urea 10.46 mmol/l (BUN 63 mg/dl); glucose 10 mmol/l (180 mg/dl); potassium 5.0 mmol/l (5.0 mEq/l).
i. What is your pre-anesthetic fluid regimen for this patient? What important factor is considered with this endocrinopathy and the cardiovascular system?
ii. Twenty-four hours after surgery and an uneventful recovery from anesthesia, suddenly the cat has repeated bouts of tetanic convulsion. What is the most likely etiology?
iii. Serum calcium is measured at 1.05 mmol/l (4.2 mg/dl). What is the immediate and long-term treatment for this condition?

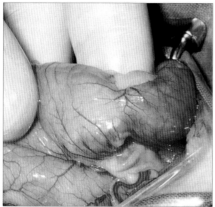

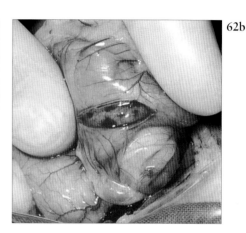

62 Two forms of chronic gastric outflow obstruction (**62a**) are encountered clinically in dogs.
i. Describe these two disorders.
ii. What breeds are commonly affected?
iii. A surgical technique used in the past to alleviate the clinical signs is shown (**62b**). Name the procedure, and the disadvantages of this technique.

63 Cyanoacrylates are used extensively as tissue adhesives.
i. List three common uses.
ii. List three applications where cyanoacrylate would not be a good choice for tissue closure.

61 i. Renal insufficiency is present. To help maintain renal perfusion during surgery, diuresis is induced with i/v administration of saline (0.9%) at 10–20 ml/kg per hour, and mannitol at 0.25–1 g/kg. This reverses arteriolar vasoconstriction, expands intravascular fluid volume and decreases renin secretion.

Hypertrophic cardiomyopathy often occurs with hyperthyroidism. Assessment of cardiac function by thoracic radiographs, electrocardiogram and echocardiogram is performed before surgery. Care is taken to prevent volume overload of the heart.

ii. Tetany from hypocalcemia occurs from iatrogenic injury to the parathyroid glands during bilateral thyroidectomy.

iii. If hypocalcemia is severe (serum calcium <1.5 mmol/l (<6 mg/dl)), supplementation with slow i/v boluses of calcium chloride or calcium gluconate (calcium gluconate 1%: 0.5–1.5ml/kg) is given to effect during tetany; the ECG is monitored concurrently for arrythmias. Calcium chloride (1 g/250 ml of maintenance fluids) is useful to maintain normal serum calcium. Calcium supplements must not be added to lactate, acetate or bicarbonate solutions since precipitates may occur. Calcium supplementation is temporary until parathyroid gland function returns, or vitamin D therapy is initiated for long-term management of hypocalcemia.

62 i. Congenital pyloric muscle hypertrophy. Luminal obstruction is caused by concentric hypertrophy of the circular smooth muscle. Clinical signs often appear shortly after weaning.

Acquired antral hypertrophy is usually encountered in small middle-aged dogs and results from hypertrophy of the circular smooth muscle, hyperplasia of the mucosa, or both.

ii. Congenital form: brachycephalic breeds, including Boston Terrier, Boxer, Bulldog. Acquired form: Lhaso Apsa, Shi Tzu, Pekinese, Poodle.

iii. Fredet–Ramsted (FR) pyloromyotomy. Neither exposure of the mucosal surface nor obtaining a full-thickness surgical biopsy is possible in this procedure. The pyloric lumen after FR pylorotomy is not significantly larger than the lumen of control dogs after a healing period of 3–4 weeks and may actually be less because of scar formation. Y–U pyloplasty more effectively enlarges the lumen, but gastric antral resection and gastroduodenal anastomosis (Billroth I) is now more commonly performed to treat this abnormality.

63 i. Monomers of cyanoacrylate are converted from a liquid to a solid state by polymerization, catalyzed by minute amounts of water on the tissue surface. Three common areas of use are oral surgery, corneal ulcer management and cutaneous incisions.

ii. Cyanocarylates are not recommended for closure of hollow organs (eg. bowel or bladder incisions), closure of fascial incisions or as a method of stabilizing fractures.

64 You are presented with a two-year-old, spayed female Beagle that has been hit by a car. After initiating shock treatment, you begin to assess her injuries more fully. Any manipulation of the pelvis or left femur causes the dog to writhe in pain and attempt to bite.

i. How will you manage this dog's pain while you continue to stabilize her and assess the full extent of her injuries?

ii. How will you manage pain during the operative and immediate postoperative period, assuming that pelvic and femoral fractures are present?

iii. How will you manage pain once you send the animal home after surgery?

65a   65b   65c

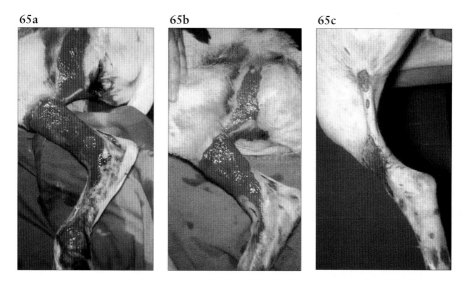

65 The open wound shown on the hindlimb of this large mixed-breed dog (65a) started as a large necrotic lesion, probably toxic epidermal necrolysis or the result of a spider bite. An outline of care was given to the owner. The wound progressed well and is shown three weeks later (65b). At this time, reconstructive surgery was recommended. The dog was not returned for further care for four months when it had developed the problem shown (65c). Most of the open wound has healed; however, the hock and stifle cannot be extended or flexed because of the tight band of scar tissue that extends from the stifle to the hock.

i. What has happened to the leg?

ii. What can be done?

64, 65: Answers

64 i. Immediate pain control is achieved by i/v administration of oxymorphone in boluses of 0.05 mg/kg each time. Wait five minutes between doses to assess the degree of pain control: stop administration of oxymorphone when the dog will allow some manipulation of the injured limb. Pain is controlled until surgery by several methods: intermittent administration of morphine (0.5–1 mg/kg i/m or s/c, q 2–6 hours) or oxymorphone (0.05–0.1 mg/kg i/v or i/m, q 3–4 hours) can be used, or more easily a transdermal fentanyl patch (50 µg/kg/hour patch) is placed on the neck under a bandage. It will take 12–18 hours for the fentanyl to reach analgesic blood concentrations, during which time tapering administration of oxymorphone or morphine can be used. The patch is active for at least three days.

ii. If a fentanyl patch was used, it will provide analgesia during surgery. Emergence delirium is pronounced with fentanyl patches and a single dose of oxymorphone (0.05 mg/kg i/v) should be given just before extubation to facilitate recovery. Alternative methods include epidural administration of a mixture of bupivacaine (0.2 ml/kg of a 0.25% solution) and morphine (0.1 mg/kg), or intermittent parenteral administration of morphine or oxymorphone.

iii. Pain can be controlled using oral drugs once the animal is sent home. Mixtures of codeine and acetaminophen are available (codeine dose of 1–2 mg/kg p/o q 6–8 hours) in several strengths and may be used unless there is evidence of liver disease. Buffered aspirin (10 mg/kg p/o q 12 hours) or carprofen (2 mg/kg p/o q 12 hours) may also be used.

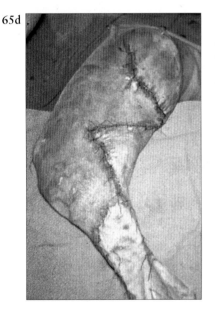

65d

65 i. This open wound has healed by contraction and epithelialization. Unfortunately, surgery was not done when recommended and further wound contraction has led to contracture deformity. The open wound on the lateral aspect of the leg above the hock has stopped contracting.

ii. The line of scar tissue is tight and inflexible. In this instance, Z-plasty will release the tension along the linear cicatricial contracture, it will change the scar from a straight line to a Z and it will bring adjacent skin into the area. An incision is made along the linear cicatricial contracture and a second and third incision are made at 60°, one on the medial side and the other on the lateral side of the leg. The resulting triangular flaps are detached and undermining is done as necessary to allow transposition of the flaps. The large open wound below the area of contracture has been grafted (**65d**). The line contracture deformity is removed and immediately there is considerable mobility in the stifle and hock.

Z-plasty is used to increase the distance between two points by bringing adjacent tissue into the central line of the Z and transforms the scar into a Z which can be stretched. The procedure is also useful to increase the circumference of a circle as in a constricted anus following perianal infections.

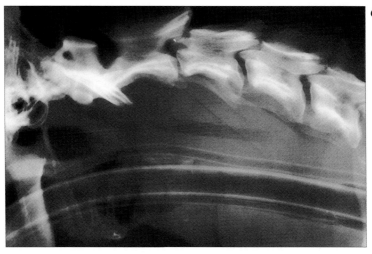

66a

66 This is a lateral radiograph (**66a**) of the cervical region in a four-year-old, male German Shepherd Dog that presented for acute onset of hypersalivation, gagging, and retching. There is no history of trauma and he is an indoor/outdoor dog with no other animals in the household.
i. Based on the history and radiograph what is the most likely diagnosis?
ii. If thoracic radiographs demonstrate pneumomediastinum, pneumothorax or pleural effusion, what has most likely happened?
iii. Describe how to resolve this problem and what complications might be encountered later?

67 i. What is the urinary apparatus shown (**67**), and what are the indications for its use?
ii. What are alternatives to use of this system?
iii. Describe the clinical management of this system.

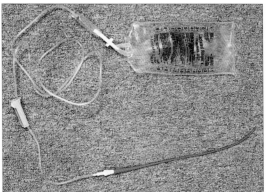

67

66b

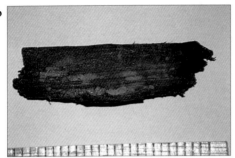

66 i. The radiograph shows a linear, radiolucent foreign body lodged in the hypaxial musculature dorsal to the cervical esophagus and ventral to the second and third cervical vertebrae. The radiopaque structure ventral to the esophagus is an endotracheal tube. The foreign body was a piece of wood (66b).
ii. If any of the above findings were evident on thoracic radiographs, tracheal perforation should be suspected.
iii. If the foreign body is protruding into the pharynx or esophagus, an attempt is made to retrieve it *per os* or by endoscopy. The area is then surgically explored for residual pieces of wood left behind. Devitalized tissues are debrided, the wound copiously lavaged, and suitable drainage is provided. If the foreign body is not visible from the pharynx, the muscles ventral to the cervical spine are explored via a ventral midline approach.

In this case the entry wound in the pharynx was not visible. The cervical hypaxial musculature was approached, the wound was cleaned and debrided, and a Penrose drain placed. This dog made a good recovery, although the general prognosis should be guarded for this problem. Foreign material is often difficult to find, and one study reported four of five dogs with lacerations of the esophagus subsequently died from mediastinitis.

If an esophageal laceration is present, tissue viability is assessed and necrotic tissue debrided. Tension-free apposition is required to achieve primary healing of the esophagus. The submucosa is the strength layer in the esophagus and there is no serosa which is important for forming a fibrin seal to prevent leakage and dehiscence. Complications of esophageal tears include dehiscence, stricture formation and infection.

67 i. This is a closed indwelling urinary drainage system made from a used i/v fluid bag, a fluid administration set and red rubber feeding tube. Polyvinyl, latex or silicone catheters can be used but stiff polyethylene catheters cause urethral damage. Foley catheters can be used in female dogs.

Indications for use of this system include: urethral obstruction; detrusor atony or dysynergia; assessment of urine production; collection of urine after chemotherapy; collection of urine from paralyzed patients; selected urethral and prostatic surgeries.
ii. Intermittent catheterization, cystocentesis or manual expression of the bladder are alternatives. Micturition is concurrently assisted by pharmacologic therapy: sphincter relaxation is promoted with phenoxybenzamine (2.5–10 mg daily) and detrusor tone is increased with bethanecol (2.5–30 mg tid).
iii. Indwelling catheters are used for the shortest possible time. The drainage system is opened using only aseptic technique, and the collection bag is never inverted or raised above the level of the bladder. Antibiotic therapy and bacterial culture are not routinely performed while the catheter is in place unless the patient shows signs of illness. Urine culture and sensitivity is performed at the time of catheter removal; appropriate antibiotic therapy is administered for 10 days.

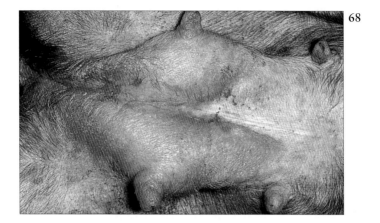

68

68 A mass on the ventrum of a 12-year-old, female, mixed-breed dog that presented after six months for evaluation of a slow growing mass (68). On palpation a hard, irregular mass is detected in the left inguinal region. The mass is approximately 12 cm long and related to the mammary tissue.
i. What is your diagnosis?
ii. What additional diagnostic or staging tests are indicated?
iii. What is the treatment?

69 This dog (69) is a six-year-old Miniature Schnauzer with a history of chronic neck pain. The dog holds its neck in a guarded position similar to patients with cervical intervertebral disc protrusion. The right mandibular lymph node is palpably enlarged.
i. What is the diagnosis?
ii. What procedure would you perform to confirm the diagnosis?
iii. What is the prognosis?

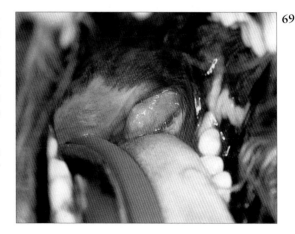

69

70 You are setting up a standardized anesthesia/analgesia protocol for performing ovariohysterectomies in dogs at a large multiveterinarian hospital.
i. Is postoperative pain control part of your protocol? Why or why not?
ii. What preoperative drugs will you recommend?

68 i. Mammary tumor. Differential diagnoses are mastitis and steatitis/cellulitis.
ii. Thoracic radiographs (ventrodorsal and both right and left lateral views) are evaluated for the presence of pulmonary metastases and screening laboratory work (hemogram, serum chemistry profile and urinalysis) for concurrent diseases. Fine-needle aspiration for cytologic analysis is not particularly helpful because of low sensitivity and specificity (97–100% and 64–78% respectively) and because 30–40% of dogs with multifocal masses will have both benign and malignant tumors. Histologic analysis is best performed on an excisional biopsy unless inflammatory carcinoma is suspected.
iii. If thoracic radiographs show no evidence of metastases, surgery is recommended. The preferred procedure is surgical resection that will result in complete excision of all cancerous tissue. This may be simple lumpectomy for a small well localized tumor, mastectomy for a larger tumor, or bilateral radical mastectomy for multiple large tumors.

If histopathologic analysis confirms neoplasia, re-examination every 3–4 months is recommended. If the tumor is malignant, thoracic radiographs (three views) are also made and adjuvant treatment with chemotherapy or radiation is considered. Fifty percent of canine mammary tumors are benign and approximately half of malignant tumors can be removed before they spread; thus effectively, a durable remission can be achieved for 75% of canine mammary tumors with early aggressive surgery. For the remaining 25% of cases, metastasis and death will occur on average within a year (range 2–24+ months).

69 i. Tonsillar squamous cell carcinoma. Patients with tonsillitis usually have bilateral tonsillar enlargement and the tonsils do not have a fleshy appearance as in this dog.
ii. Classification using the TNM system as in **19** with the principle diagnostic test being excisional biopsy of the tonsil.
iii. The prognosis for this disease is poor. With surgical excision alone, survival is often <2 months. Radiation therapy following surgical resection improved survival times to 4–5 months but most dogs still died of distant metastases.

70 i. Drugs to control postoperative pain are not traditionally used after ovariohysterectomy in dogs. Most dogs appear to recover quickly after this surgery and analgesics are not thought to be needed. In blind studies comparing the postoperative recovery of dogs undergoing ovariohysterectomy with or without analgesics, dogs treated scored lower on pain scales and had more rapid return of normal behavior. A good guide is that if a procedure is painful for humans, it is assumed to be painful for animals and analgesic drugs should be used.
ii. Pain is controlled better by prevention, than by treatment after exposure. Preoperative drugs that act as both analgesics and sedatives include morphine (0.5 mg/kg s/c), oxymorphone (0.05 mg/kg i/v, i/m or s/c) and butorphanol (0.4 mg/kg i/v, i/m or s/c). Carprofen, a non-steroidal anti-inflammatory drug, acts as an analgesic and provides good pain control after ovariohysterectomy. The dose is 4 mg/kg p/o once, one hour before surgery.

71 With regard to the protocol for performing ovariohysterectomies in dogs at the large multiveterinarian hospital in question **70**:
i. How will you monitor for postoperative pain?
ii. What postoperative pain control therapy will you recommend?

72 i. A steam sterilized pack, double wrapped in Quarpel treated 270 pima cloth, is considered sterile for how long?
ii. How is this time altered if the pack is wrapped in paper?
iii. How is the time altered if ethylene oxide sterilization is used?

73 This is a skull radiograph of a five-year-old, male German Shepherd Dog that presented for chronic sanguinopurulent nasal discharge, ulceration of the external nares and intermittent epistaxis (**73**).
i. Based on this radiograph, what is the diagnosis and what signs enable you to be confident of your diagnosis?
ii. What other diagnostic tests would be useful to perform?
iii. Describe the most non-invasive treatment for this condition. Why does this therapy provide a better prognosis, and what complications can occur?

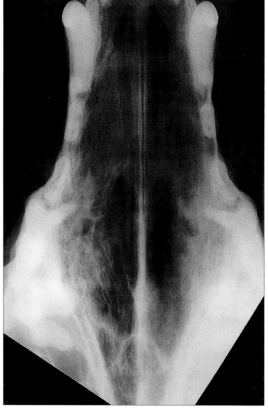

73

61

71 i. Veterinarians traditionally use gross behavioral evidence of pain (vocalization, vocalization on manipulation, lameness, refusal to move, obvious difficulty in rising, etc.) to monitor animals. These signs occur when the animal has reached the extreme limits of pain tolerance. Healthy animals not given analgesics after ovariohysterectomy display much more subtle evidence of pain: they raise their lip slightly on palpation, they stay awake the night after surgery, and they do not come to the front of the cage and wag their tails when someone approaches. High heart rates after surgery may be due to pain, but are more often related to cardiovascular instability.
ii. Morphine (1 mg/kg i/m or s/c, q 2–6 hours), oxymorphone (0.05 mg/kg i/v, i/m or s/c, q 3–4 hours) and butorphanol (0.4 mg/kg i/v, i/m or s/c, q 1–2 hours) all provide analgesia. The sedative effects of butorphanol last longer than the analgesic effects, which confounds patient monitoring. Carprofen does not need to be redosed until 12 hours after surgery. Flunixin meglumine (0.5–1.0 mg/kg i/v once) may be used for pain control after surgery in healthy dogs, but should not be used preoperatively due to increased risk of inducing renal compromise during surgery.

72 i. Forty nine days in an enclosed cabinet or 21 days on an open shelf.
ii. The time is extended to 56 days minimum in a cabinet and remains 21 days on an open shelf.
iii. It is shortened to 15–30 days for cloth and 30–60 days for paper wraps. Plastic wraps extend safe storage times to 90–100 days if tape sealed and up to one year if heat sealed.

73 i. Mycotic rhinitis due to *Aspergillus* spp. *(A. fumigatus* is the most common isolate) or *Penicillium* spp. is typical of the pattern present on radiographs. There is marked turbinate destruction and an overall radiolucency of the left nasal chamber. Other diagnostic considerations include intranasal foreign body (although increased opacity is commonly seen around the object) and neoplasia (aggressive destruction of turbinates, vomer bone and/or facial bones is seen, but usually with a homogeneous increase in opacity of the nasal passages).
ii. Rhinoscopy may reveal white, yellow or green fungal plaques on the nasal mucosa; concurrent biopsy samples are taken for histologic analysis, culture and cytologic examination. Serologic testing is performed (AGID or ELISA) but cross-reactivity between *Aspergillus* spp. and *Penicillium* spp. may make them hard to differentiate by this method.
iii. Treatment of nasal aspergillosis is by infusion of enilconazole or clotrimazole through an 8 French polypropylene catheter placed through the external nares midway along the dorsal nasal meatus on each side. The nares and nasopharynx are occluded using gauze sponges or laparotomy pads and the dog is placed in dorsal recumbency. After injection of the agent, the animal is placed in ventral recumbency and the nose tipped to allow drainage of excess fluid. Complications of this procedure include recurrence from incomplete distribution of the antifungal agent (although less likely to occur than with the surgical technique), and aspiration pneumonia or esophagitis from leakage of the agent if occlusion of the nasopharynx is not performed properly.

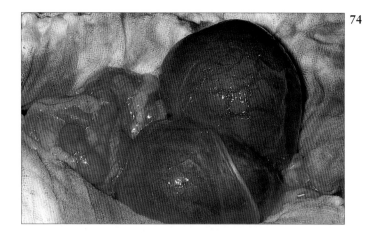

74

74 The figure (74) shows an eight-year-old male dog at exploratory surgery. The mass adjacent to the bladder was thin walled and filled with clear yellow fluid. There were several adhesions to the prostate, but an anatomic communication with the gland was not identified.
i. What is the most likely diagnosis?
ii. What anatomic structure is thought to be involved in this process?
iii. What are the surgical treatments for this abnormality, and what are the advantages and disadvantages of each?

75 Match the hemostatic forceps illustrated (75) with their intended use.
i. Control of small bleeding vessels.
ii. Control of large bleeding vessels.
iii. Control of large bleeding vessels and ligation of a large pedicle.

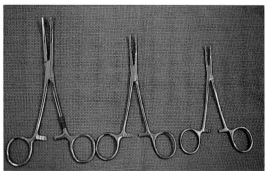

75

76 A swelling is present on the neck of a three-year-old, male cat that was bitten by another cat two days previously. The swelling is turgid and marked pain is present on palpation.
i. How would you treat this wound?
ii. Is it necessary to have any kind of postsurgical drainage? Why or why not?
iii. If you were to use a drain for this case, what are the basic rules of drain placement?

74–76: Answers

74 i. Periprostatic cyst. The size of the cyst and the absence of communication with the prostate make this the most probable diagnosis.
ii. Periprostatic cysts are thought to arise from the uterus masculinus, a remnant of the Müllerian duct system. Serosal cysts and hemorrhage can also result in periprostatic cyst formation.
iii. Cyst resection is curative if the origin is identified. Disadvantages include more extensive prostatic manipulation needed to identify the origin of the cyst and recurrence in the case of inadequate resection. A recent report described good success using omentalization of the cyst remnant after subtotal resection.

Marsupialization provides continuous drainage, and prostatic manipulation is minimized reducing the likelihood of damage to the prostatic neurovascular supply. The cyst is anchored to the paramedian rectus abdominus muscle. The cyst membrane is incised and the fluid drained and cultured. The cyst wall is then sutured to the skin to form a semi-permanent stoma. Disadvantages include difficulty in mobilizing the cyst to reach the abdominal wall and prolonged drainage. Resection is required if the cyst cannot be mobilized sufficiently. The stoma usually closes spontaneously by eight weeks postoperatively. Biopsy of the prostate and cyst wall and castration are performed at the time of resection or marsupialization to identify neoplasia and prevent recurrence of prostatic disease by inducing involution.

75 i. Halsted mosquito forceps (right).
ii. Kelly hemostatic forceps (center).
iii. Rochester–Carmalt forceps (left). These are the hemostatic forceps most commonly used in veterinary surgery. Mosquito forceps are suitable only for control of small bleeding vessels and are not designed for clamping large vessels or bundles of tissue. Kelly forceps are slightly larger than mosquito forceps and are designed for ligation of medium sized vessels. Rochester–Carmalt forceps are designed for ligation of large tissue pedicles and vessels, and have longitudinal grooves that prevent tissues from slipping through the clamp under traction. Improper use of tissue forceps leads to failure at the box lock. This may be tested by lightly rapping the instrument on a surface; a functioning box lock will not spring open whereas an improperly functioning box lock will.

76 i. The abscess is lanced and drained, and the wound lavaged and debrided. Lacerations should be sutured closed and drainage maintained for 3–5 days.
ii. Drainage must be established. This is an infected wound with a large amount of necrotic cellular debris. Wound healing cannot progress beyond the inflammatory phase until wound debris is eliminated by surgical debridement or host phagocytes.
iii. Drains must span the extent of dead space created by the wound. The smallest and fewest number of drains necessary are used for the shortest possible time. For non-suction drains, the exit end of the drain must be dependant to facilitate gravity flow and prevent pooling in the wound space. Drains should not enter or exit through a suture line; they are placed through separate stab incisions. Conduit drains (e.g. Penrose) should not be fenestrated. Fluid flow is related to surface area and fenestrations decrease surface area and hence fluid flow. In contaminated areas (e.g. perineum) the clinician must bear in mind that drains provide a venue for contaminant transport both out of *and* into a wound. Drain openings are managed aseptically, clipped free of hair and cleaned daily.

77 This ten-year-old cat presents with signs of gastrointestinal obstruction (77a). An exploratory laparotomy is performed and a jejunal mass is found. A fine-needle aspiration biopsy is performed and microscopic evaluation reveals neoplastic epithelial cells often forming acini.
i. What is your diagnosis, and what are the differential diagnoses?
ii. What diagnostic tests could be used to confirm the preliminary diagnosis?
iii. Name a breed that is reported to be commonly affected, and what is the prognosis for this type of tumor?

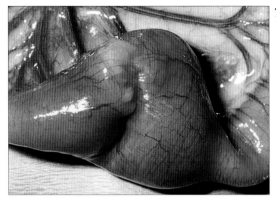
77a

78 Clinical signs for this dog (78) include halitosis and reluctance to eat or drink.
i. What is the diagnosis?
ii. What are the possible etiologies for this lesion?
iii. What would be an appropriate treatment plan?

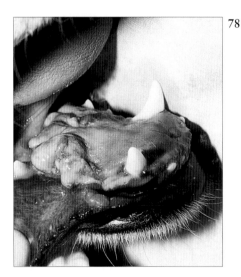
78

79 You are planning to repair a ruptured cruciate ligament in a ten-year-old, spayed female Golden Retriever. She is at least 7 kg overweight.
i. What local technique might you use to control pain after surgery?
ii. What systemic drugs do you plan to use after surgery?
iii. Will the use of analgesics make the dog more likely to use the leg prematurely after surgery, endangering your repair?

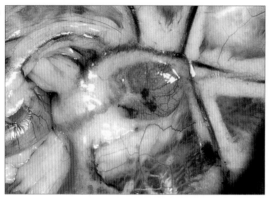

77b

77 i. Differential diagnoses include malignant lymphoma, adenocarcinoma, mast cell tumor, leiomyoma and leiomyosarcoma. Based on the description given, adenocarcinoma is most likely, although lymphoma is the most common tumor type in cats.
ii. Histologic evaluation of frozen or formalin-fixed biopsy material of the tumor and enlarged lymph nodes.
iii. Siamese cats. More than 70% of cats with intestinal adenocarcinoma have gross or histologic evidence of metastatic disease at the time of diagnosis. In cats the most common abdominal metastatic sites are abdominal serosa, lymph nodes (77b), lung and liver. However, average survival times up to 15 months are reported after complete surgical excision.

78 i. Oral mucosa and gingival necrosis.
ii. Thermal, chemical or electrical trauma.
iii. Attempt to determine any other systemic manifestations of the trauma such as pulmonary edema (electrical) or esophageal dysfunction (chemical). Superficial debridement of devitalized mucosa. If vitality is in doubt, do not resect; the dead tissue will slough. Warm water lavage performed by the owner will aid debridement. If the patient does not eat, consider placement of a nasoesophageal feeding tube or percutaneous endoscopic gastrostomy tube. Monitoring of bone and dental integrity using physical and radiographic examination will aid determination of delayed effects on other tissues. Finally, check the maxilla for associated lesions.

79 i. Placing 0.5 ml/kg of a 0.5% bupivacaine solution in the joint at the conclusion of the repair is an effective method of reducing pain after cruciate surgery in the dog.
ii. Carprofen, morphine, oxymorphone or butorphanol would each provide some degree of analgesia after surgery. Buprenorphine (0.005–0.02 mg/kg i/v or i/m, q 4–12 hours) might also be used.
iii. Analgesic therapy may result in early postoperative use of the limb. If the limb is painful, the animal is less likely to place weight on the limb. However, pain can also make the dog step awkwardly on the limb, which could also strain the repair. If the dog appeared inclined to be overly active after surgery, judicious use of tranquilizers would be a more humane method of enforcing rest than pain.

80 A 12-year-old, castrated male Kees-hound dog presents with hypercalcemia and calcium oxalate uroliths (see 50) and is diagnosed with primary hyperparathyroidism. Exploratory surgery of the cervical region was performed and a parathyroid adenoma (80) was found – the hemostat is pointing to the enlarged cranial parathyroid gland. The other parathyroid glands were too small to be identified during surgery. The enlarged parathyroid gland was surgically excised.

i. What are the benefits and risks of resection for a parathyroid adenoma?

ii. How is hypocalcemic tetany treated and how can one prevent severe hypocalcemia from developing after parathyroidectomy?

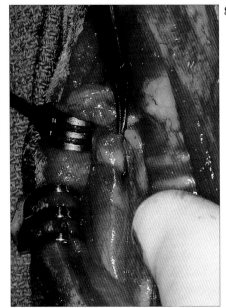

80

81 A dog presented for lethargy, tenesmus and inappetence. A diagnosis of prostatic abscess was made on the basis of the physical examination, hemogram, serum chemistry analysis, urinalysis and ultrasound examination. At surgery pus was readily aspirated from the enlarged gland (81).

i. Name four surgical treatments for this disease.

ii. What are the complications of the listed surgical treatments?

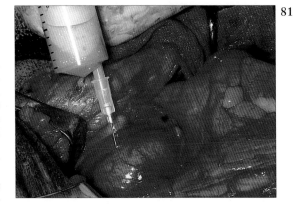

81

iii. What other surgical procedures are indicated in addition to management of the abscess?

80 i. Surgical excision of a parathyroid adenoma results in rapid resolution of hypercalcemia, and is considered curative in most cases. The most serious complication associated with the removal is postoperative hypocalcemia. The remaining parathyroid glands are atrophied due to the negative feedback of chronic persistent hypercalcemia.

ii. Hypocalcemia generally occurs within the first week after surgery. Tetanic convulsions are treated on an emergency basis with administration of calcium gluconate (0.5–1.5 ml/kg i/v administered slowly over a period of 15–30 minutes). To prevent hypocalcemia, vitamin D and calcium is supplemented after surgery. Dihydrotachysterol (0.03 mg/kg/day p/o for two days, then 0.02 mg/kg/day for two days and then 0.01 mg/kg/day) is the vitamin D supplement most often used due to its quick onset of action. Calcium is supplemented at a dose in dogs of 1–4 g/day p/o divided and in cats of 0.5–1 g/day p/o divided. Calcium concentrations are re-evaluated weekly until the remaining parathyroid glands resume their normal productivity.

81 i. The surgical treatments are:

• Partial prostatectomy/abscess resection.
• Penrose tube drainage.
• Prostatic omentalization.
• Total prostatectomy.

ii. Complications of surgical treatment for prostatic abscess include sepsis, reabscessation, urethral rupture and fistula formation, hemorrhage, and urinary incontinence. Dogs with prostatic abscessation are often septic and surgical manipulations can cause rupture and further release of bacteria and endotoxin into the peritoneum. Early identification, prompt treatment and intraoperative containment of pus and fluid is important to minimize morbidity and mortality.

Partial prostatectomy is effective if the abscess is focal. Resection results in a low incidence of incontinence, reabscessation and urethral rupture. However, the majority of prostatic abscesses are diffuse and not easily amenable to resection, and if an animal is septic at the time of surgery, this technique can be time consuming and more risky to the patient.

Penrose tube drainage can be performed rapidly providing a decided advantage when considering anesthesia of the septic patient. Recurrences are most common with drainage, and rupture of the prostatic urethra during drain placement and urethral fistulae formation are potential complications. Incontinence is least common with prostatic drain techniques.

Prostatic omentalization is as effective as prostatectomy in preventing recurrence and has a very low incidence of postoperative complications. In this technique an omental flap is passed around the urethra through the prostatic parenchymal abscess to provide additional blood and lymphatic supply and serve as a biologic drain. Because the surgeon must dissect dorsal to the urethra, care is taken to prevent urethral rupture.

Prostatectomy is very successful in preventing recurrence and urethral rupture, but has an unacceptably high incidence of postoperative incontinence (up to 90%).

iii. Two procedures are performed as additional management of prostatic abscess: biopsy is necessary because multiple prostatic diseases can occur concomitantly (e.g. abscess and neoplasia); castration is performed because prostatic hypertrophy and secretions are androgen stimulated.

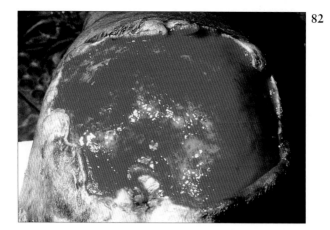

82

82 The dorsal perineum and caudal lumbar regions of a Cocker Spaniel is shown (82). Surgical and mechanical (bandage) debridement were used to treat a non-healing, infected bite wound.
i. What is the name and composition of the red exposed tissues?
ii. How could this wound be reduced for progressive healing to occur?

83 There are three layers in the construction of a typical bandage. Briefly describe the layers and their function, and give a specific example or two of each layer type.

84 A three-year-old, female English Bulldog (84) is presented for suspected dystocia. It is 67 days since the first breeding and 65 days since the second. On examination the dog has marked mammary enlargement with minimal milk production, and a distended abdomen. No other abnormalities are noted.
i. Give several causes of dystocia.
ii. Does this dog have primary or secondary uterine inertia?
iii. What is the treatment, given your diagnosis?

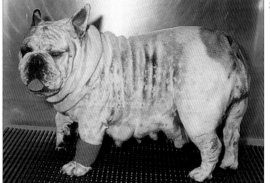

84

82 i. A healthy bleeding bed of granulation tissue which is composed of capillary and lymph vessels, fibroblasts, small amounts of collagen and macrophages. This tissue serves as a barrier against infection, a bed for epithelialization and a source for wound contraction and support. Granulation tissue is the hallmark of the repair stage or second phase of wound healing.

ii. With a healthy granulation bed present, wound closure is easily achieved using free skin grafts (usually meshed) or neighboring pedicle skin flaps. Granulation tissue is highly resistant to infection and provides a ready source for neovascularization, enhancing the survival of transposed tissue.

83 Primary layer (material apposed to the wound) – can be used to debride tissue or provide a non-stick surface for wound granulation and epithelialization. The primary layer should wick fluid away from the wound to the secondary layer, be semi-permeable to moisture and oxygen, and conform to the wound surface. Primary bandage layers include: saline soaked gauze pads as used in a wet-to-dry bandage, and petroleum impregnated gauze as used in a non-stick bandage. Secondary layer (middle layer) is used for absorption, padding, or rigid support. The most common secondary layer is cotton, and different thicknesses can be applied depending on the desired function. Splint material (plastic, metal, fiberglass, etc.) is incorporated into this layer for immobilization. Tertiary layer (outside covering of bandage) for protection from the environment. Ideally it is rugged enough to withstand wear and tear initiated by the animal, and provides some degree of water resistance. For each layer the ideal bandage material should be easy to apply, wrapping around contours with good fit, be non-toxic to tissues preventing delayed wound healing, and be cost effective to use.

84 i. Dystocia is considered when: a bitch shows signs of toxicity or exhaustion; 20 minutes of strong labor or 2–3 hours of weak labor has failed to produce a puppy; more than four hours has elapsed between puppies; there is abnormal vulvar discharge; or there is prolonged gestation of more than 70 days. Causes include primary uterine inertia (lack of sufficient uterine contractions to expel a normal fetus from a normal birth canal) and secondary uterine inertia (lack of sufficient contractions because of exhaustion from prolonged labor or metabolic abnormality). Secondary inertia is caused by maternal factors (e.g. vulvar or pelvic obstruction; uterine torsion or rupture; and uncommonly from hypocalcemia or hypoglycemia), and by fetal factors such as oversize fetuses (commonly with small litters and brachycephalic breeds), congenital disorders (e.g monster puppies and hydrocephalus), fetal malpositioning and dead fetuses.

ii. This dog does not have dystocia at this time. While the average bitch whelps around 63 days from the time of breeding, gestational length is variable ranging from 56–72 days. This dog has shown no clinical signs of active labor or whelping abnormality ruling out secondary inertia as a problem and has not yet exceeded the gestational time range considered normal for ruling out primary uterine inertia.

iii. Treatment is nothing more than close observation over the next few days for signs of whelping. Rectal temperature is monitored: less than 37.7°C (100°F) indicates declining serum progesterone concentration and impending parturition (usually within 24 hours). If fetal viability is suspect, radiographs or sonography are performed. After 69–70 days from the time of the second breeding (or ideally LH peak), primary uterine inertia is considered present, and diagnosis and treatment for dystocia initiated.

85 An eight-month-old Weimaraner is presented with signs of ileus. The cause of the ileus is shown (85a).
i. What is the clinical diagnosis, and what are predisposing factors?
ii. Name in decreased order of frequency the most common sites for occurrence of this disease process.
iii. What surgical technique is reported to prevent recurrence of this disease process?

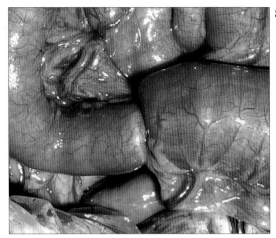
85a

86 When considering interventional nutritional support for a surgery patient, what are the relevant points for deciding the route of feeding?

87 An ulcerating lesion of approximately two years duration on the back of a four-year-old Doberman Pinscher is shown (87). Many unsuccessful attempts were made to close this defect and biopsies were taken to rule out neoplasia. The lesion originally extended down both flanks and the present size is the result of wound contraction. Scar tissue is palpated extending into the flanks and the skin surrounding the lesion is extremely tight.
i. What reconstructive procedures can be considered to correct this abnormality?

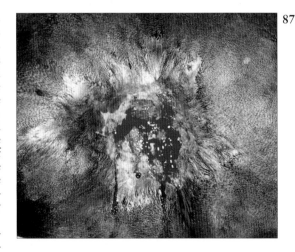
87

ii. After alternatives are considered, a decision is made to use a tissue expander. What is the physiologic mechanism by which this device provides sufficient skin to cover a defect?

85b

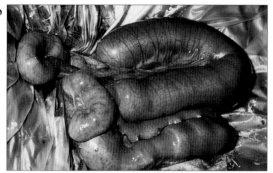

85 i. Intussusception. Abnormal intestinal motility caused by viral and bacterial infections; intestinal parasitism; and acute inflammatory disorders including neoplasia, diverticula, and chronic infiltrative disease may predispose to intussusception formation.
ii. Ileocolic junction, ileum, jejunum, cecum and duodenum.
iii. Enteroplication of the jejunum and ileum (85b). The intestine is folded into loops from the distal duodenum to distal ileum. The lateral borders of each loop are sutured to the adjacent loop with simple interrupted monofilament suture material.

86 Feeding should be as close to physiologically normal as the affecting disease process allows. If an animal will tolerate oral feeding (forced or drug stimulated), it is best used. The disadvantage is that adequate intake is difficult to maintain in an anorectic animal; they do not readily tolerate forced feeding and effective drug stimulation is usually transient. Drug stimulation is best for cases of partial anorexia. If vomiting is not occurring and oral intake is inadequate, esophageal or gastric tube feeding (e.g. nasogastric, pharyngostomy, esophagostomy, gastrostomy) is indicated. With most of these methods (except nasogastric tube) a large bore tube is placed for administration into the stomach. Hyperosmotic, calorie-dense diets can be used, and intermittent feeding is tolerated because of the stomach's reservoir effect. The disadvantage is that anesthesia is required to place some feeding devices (pharyngostomy and gastrostomy tubes). If vomiting is present, a jejunostomy feeding tube is needed. Disadvantages are that surgical placement is needed and, because of the smaller tube bore and enteric administration, continuous infusion of isosmotic liquid diets is required. If malabsorption is present or anesthesia is not feasible, parenteral nutrition is needed. The disadvantage is the high cost and labor intensiveness of parenteral feeding.

87 i. Skin surrounding this wound is exceptionally tight so local skin mobilization is not possible. Skin grafting is avoided on the body because of problems with immobilization. An axial pattern flap using the deep circumflex iliac vessels can be used to cover the lesion, but is not selected because of possible involvement of these vessels in the original wound. Use of a tissue expander and single pedicle advancement flap is preferred.
ii. Skin is capable of expanding over slowly enlarging masses (e.g. tumor or an enlarging abdomen). Controversy exists but evidence is that mitotic activity occurs in the epidermis and that it retains its original thickness; the dermis and panniculus carnosus muscle, however, become thinner. When skin over the expander is harvested for transfer, the thick fibrous capsule which forms over the expander is transferred with the epidermis and dermis to restore the original thickness. Skin can necrose, especially over bone, if the expander is filled too rapidly. Skin flaps created by expansion have improved survival when compared to acutely raised flaps because of the 'delay phenomenon' (if blood circulation to skin is compromised, collateral or remaining vessels expand in response).

88 With regard to the tissue expander discussed in **87**, how is this device used? How rapidly is the expander distended? When is the final surgical procedure done?

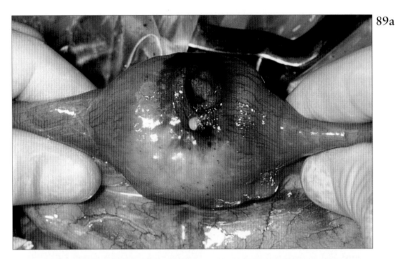

89a

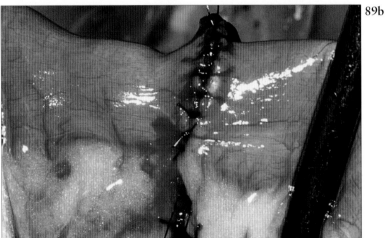

89b

89 A two-year-old, mixed-breed dog is presented with a two-day history of vomiting and diarrhea. A jejunal foreign body is found during abdominal exploratory surgery (**89a**). The foreign body is removed by intestinal resection and end-to-end anastomosis (**89b**).
i. Describe four suture techniques for end-to-end anastomosis.
ii. Name the major disadvantage of each technique.
iii. What are the advantages and disadvantages of stapling techniques?

73

88a

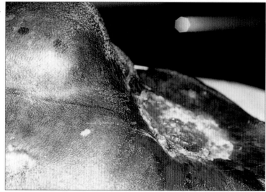

88b

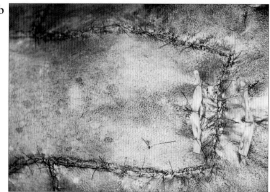

88 The expander device includes an inflatable bag (expander) connected by tube to a dome-shaped filling reservoir. Expander size and shape can vary, and ready-made and customized expanders are available. The expander is surgically placed close to the recipient area, and the incision is made with care so that it does not interfere with the final donor flap. The filling reservoir is placed distant to the expander to avoid becoming covered and inaccessible for needle puncture. The dome of the filling reservoir is easily palpable under the skin.

The expander is filled with saline slowly over six weeks or more. In acute wounds there are practical difficulties. In one experimental report, expanders were filled in seven days and skin flaps were harvested. There were some negative effects and more investigation is needed.

In this dog the expander was filled once weekly, using no sedation or analgesia, with approximately 60 ml of sterile normal saline. The filled expander containing approximately 360 ml of saline is shown at six weeks (88a). Lines are shown on the skin to indicate the incisions of a single pedicle advancement flap utilizing the loose skin made available. The finished flap is shown (88b).

89 i. Inverting, everting, crushing and approximating suture patterns.
ii. Inverting suture pattern: decrease of luminal size. Everting suture pattern: increase in incidence of adhesion formation. Crushing suture pattern: increase in tissue necrosis and disruption of blood vessels during the first week after surgery. Appositional technique: mucosal eversion between sutures.
iii. The advantages of stapling techniques include greater speed, greater blood flow through the anastomosis, greater bursting strength and less inflammatory reaction compared to certain suture techniques. Stapling equipment is more expensive compared with conventional suturing techniques.

90 An exploratory laparotomy in a two-year-old German Shepherd Dog with a history of intermittent hematochezia and soft stools is shown (90a).
i. What is your diagnosis?
ii. What breed predilection has been suggested, and what etiology has been suspected to play a role in the pathogenesis?
iii. What diagnostic test should be performed?
iv. What is the surgical therapy?

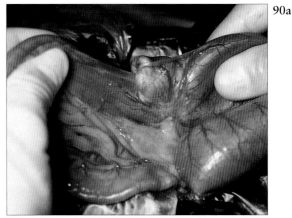

91 This is a one-year-old, female Terrier-mix breed presented for intermittent dribbling since its acquisition at three months of age (91). This dog periodically voids the bladder normally.
i. What diagnosis is suggested by the contrast study?
ii. What are five morphologic variations of this anatomic anomaly?
iii. What are the methods of choice for assessing the ureteral pathway and its termination?

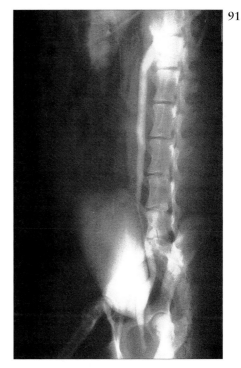

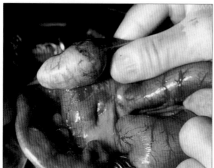
90b

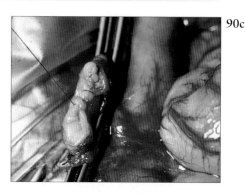
90c

90 i. Partial cecal inversion (90b).
ii. Young, large-breed, male dogs are pre-disposed. Weimaraner dogs are suggested to have a higher risk. *Trichuris* worms are reported to be a causative agent.
iii. Plain abdominal radiographs often are not diagnostic. Pneumocolonography and colonoscopy are more successful in determining the diagnosis.
iv. Typhlectomy is the treatment of choice for a partial cecal inversion (90c, d). Total cecal inversion is treated by surgical resection of the ileocolic junction.

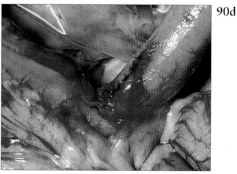
90d

91 i. The excretory urogram shows ureteral ectopia; here the dilated left ureter drains into the urethra. It is a congenital disorder where one (70–80% of dogs) or both ureters (most cats) terminate and drain at a site other than the urinary bladder, most often in the urethra or vagina. The condition occurs most frequently in Siberian Huskies, Newfoundlands, Terriers, Golden and Labrador Retrievers and Toy Poodles; the mode of inheritance is unknown.
ii. The five morphologic variations of this anatomic anomaly are:

• Intramural ureter with the opening distal to the bladder sphincter. This is the most common type of ectopic ureter.
• Intramural ureter with no distal opening.
• Intramural ureter with two distal openings – one above and one below the bladder sphincter.
• Intramural ureter with a normal opening and a ureteral trough continuing distal to the sphincter.
• Extramural ureter that enters directly into the vagina or urethra without penetrating the bladder wall.

iii. An excretory urogram in conjunction with pneumocystogram is useful to assess the presence or absence of an ectopic ureter. Vagino-urethrography is also useful for evaluating the termination of the ureter. Radiography cannot be used to identify the morphologic type of ectopic ureter.

92 The dog shown (**92**) had an esophagotomy for removal of a bone. There was mild esophageal mucosal hemorrhage and erosion but the muscular tunic was intact. There was no evidence of esophageal perforation.

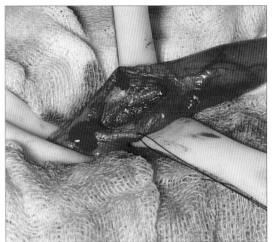

92

i. What is the most appropriate suture pattern for closure of the esophagotomy wound?
ii. What is the holding layer of the esophagus?
iii. If the incision margins have questionable viability, what options exist for reinforcement of the incision?

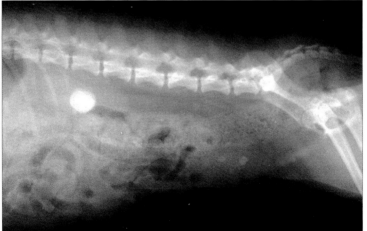

93a

93 A lateral abdominal radiograph of a five-year-old, male Beagle is shown (**93a**). Diagnostic evaluation of this dog identified pylonephritis (urine culture grew *Escherichia coli*) and mild azotemia (urea 6.97 mmol/l (BUN 42 mg/dl)), urine specific gravity 1,020). Surgical removal of the calculi is planned.
i. Which surgical technique is least deleterious to renal function?
ii. If the technique from (**i.**) is not applicable, which technique is most commonly used? What are the consequences on renal function?
iii. What should be thought of less invasive procedures such as lithotripsy for animals?

92 i. The ideal suture pattern is easily performed, sufficiently strong to resist dehiscence, provides a watertight seal, does not result in stricture and provides anatomic alignment of the tissues. This is best accomplished by a double layer simple interrupted suture pattern in the submucosa/mucosa and the muscularis/adventitia. Simple interrupted single layer closure has similar strength and can be performed more quickly, but provides poor anatomic alignment of tissues. Simple continuous patterns are placed quickly and have similar ultimate (28 day) wound strength, but result in poor anatomic alignment of tissues and inhibit luminal distension.

ii. The submucosa contains the most collagen and is therefore the holding layer of the esophagus. Previously, several investigators maintained that the mucosa was the holding layer of the esophagus because it is thicker and has a substantial lamina propria. Sutures in the submucosa have equal tensile strength to mucosal/submucosal sutures and comparable strength to full thickness sutures.

iii. A vascularized omental or pericardial flap can be used to deliver blood and lymphatic supply to the esophageal wound and to bridge defects. Muscular reinforcement of esophageal anastomosis using the sternohyoideus (cervical esophagus) or pedicled intercostal muscle (thoracic esophagus) can be used; the disadvantage is decreased distensibility and they cannot be used to bridge esophageal defects.

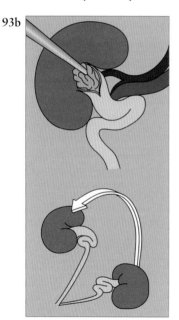

93b

93 i. If renal calculi are within a dilated proximal ureter or the extra-renal portion of the renal pelvis, a dorsal pyelolithotomy is preferred (**93b**). Advantages of this technique are that there is no destruction of nephrons and it does not require renal vascular occlusion because the surgical incision is made in the pelvis rather than through renal parenchyma.

ii. When calculi are deep into the renal pelvis or when there are many small calculi, bisection nephrotomy allows better visualization of the renal pelvis and diverticulae facilitating removal of stones. Disadvantages are destruction of functional nephrons (patients are often azotemic) and more prolific hemorrhage than pylolithotomy (patients are often anemic). Hemostasis is improved by obstructing the renal artery with a bulldog vascular clamp (occlusion should not exceed 20 minutes). Bisection nephrotomy decreases renal function in operated kidneys by 30–50% (direct incisional effect, indirect devascularization) and transfixing sutures further compromise glomerular filtration rate. Intersegmental nephrotomy offers no significant protective effect for preservation of kidney function. In the case of advanced pyelonephritis or hydronephrosis, ureteronephrectomy is recommended.

iii. Lithotripsy is not currently an option in companion animals given the relative hardness of the stones, the risk for kidney and lung parenchyma damage and the prohibitive cost and inaccessibility of equipment. Experimental percutaneous nephrolithotomy has been described in the dog but is not yet clinically practical.

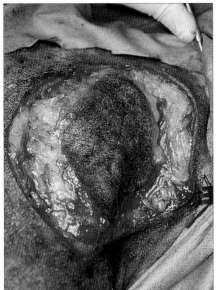

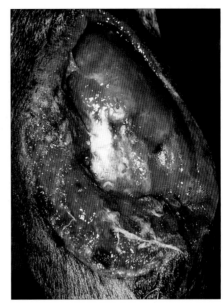

94 The wound illustrated (94a) resulted from removal of a mast cell tumor in a dog. There is ample skin for closure of the defect.
i. Name three suture techniques that can be used to repair this circular wound.
ii. Placement of the initial sutures resulted in a 'dog ear'. List three methods of correcting this fold.

95 The stifle joint area of a Labrador Retriever treated three months earlier for a cranial cruciate ligament injury is shown (95). The limb is non-functional and an open, draining wound has been present for nearly a month.
i. How would this wound be classified with respect to contamination?
ii. What are the treatment options and prognosis?

96 A cat is presented two days after being hit by a car. Although recovering rapidly from initial hypovolemic shock, the cat's condition has been deteriorating for 24 hours. The 13th rib is fractured on the left side. Gross hematuria is present and serum urea nitrogen is elevated. Abdominal radiographs show good peritoneal contrast; however, the left retroperitoneal area is opaque and the kidney not readily visible.
i. What diagnoses are suspected?
ii. Which clinical tests will likely lead to a definitive diagnosis?

94–96: Answers

94b

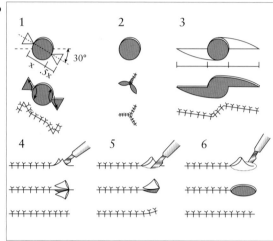

94 i. Create a fusiform defect by removing triangles of skin from opposite edges of the circle (1.5 times the diameter of the circle) (**94b**, 1). The incision is then closed with simple interrupted sutures. This is an excellent technique but is restricted to areas where there is ample skin for reconstruction.The wound may be closed with a three point intradermal suture to create a Y-shaped defect (**94b**, 2). Each leg of the Y is closed with simple inter-rupted sutures. This closure may result in 'dog ears' that must be addressed.

O to Z closure may be used when closure under tension or deviation of tissues will have adverse consequences (e.g. around the nares or eyes) (**94b**, 3). With this technique, curvilinear incisions are made in opposite directions on opposite sides of the circle. The resulting flaps are undermined and brought together to result in a Z-shaped closure.
ii. The skin incision may be extended through the 'dog ear' and two triangles of affected skin removed (**94b**, 4); incision along the base of one 'dog ear' and extension of the incision through the 'dog ear' (removal of the resulting skin triangle results in a curved end to the incision) (**94b**, 5); extension of a fusiform incision to include the affected skin with closure of the defect routinely (**94b**, 6).

95 i. The surgical incision has undergone dehiscence. This wound is a chronic, open, dirty lesion consisting of excessive granulation tissue, exposed bone and necrotic purulent debris.
ii. Surgical treatment is by tissue debridement, wound lavage, removal of infected lateral imbricating sutures, and partial closure to reduce contamination and permit evaluation of granulation tissue formation. Because of potential joint involvement by the wound, broad-spectrum bactericidal antibiotics are administered based on culture and sensitivity testing. Prognosis for normal recovery is poor due to the chronic and severe nature of the joint injury.

96 i. Hemo- or uroretroperitoneum is likely. At this point, a ureteral tear cannot be distinguished from renal or other retroperitoneal trauma.
ii. Excretory urography is the diagnostic test of choice to diagnose and distinguish renal versus ureteral trauma. Look for an accumulation of contrast material in the area of suspected leakage. Iodine-based contrast is administered intravenously (325 mg iodine/kg) and radiographs are taken at 0, 5 and 10 minutes. Ultrasonography may be helpful to delineate renal integrity. Pulsed Doppler echography can help determine whether renal arteries are patent, and is less invasive than renal arteriography.

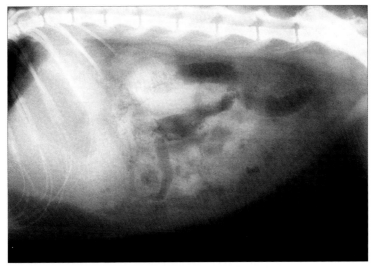

97a

97 This is a right lateral abdominal radiograph of a nine-year-old, domestic short-hair cat (97a). Clinical signs included fever, vomiting, depression, anorexia and diarrhea for two days. Pain is elicited by palpation of all areas of the abdomen.
i. Describe your radiographic interpretation and most likely diagnosis.
ii. What diagnostic tests should be performed, and what is their accuracy?
iii. Intracellular bacteria are found on cytologic analysis of the abdominal fluid. An exploratory laparotomy is performed and the colon is found to be ruptured. The colon is resected. What technique is used to establish effective peritoneal cavity drainage, and what is the prognosis?

98 Describe four types of restraint devices to prevent animals from traumatizing themselves, their bandages or other surgical appliances.

99 Digit III on the right rear foot of a ten-year-old, female German Shepherd Dog is enlarged. The owners first noticed the toe was swollen approximately four weeks prior to presentation. In the interim time the swelling has increased in size and a small ulcerative area has developed on the medial surface of the digit. On palpation the digit is moderately firm and the popliteal lymph node is enlarged and firm. A radiograph of the foot shows lysis of the third pharynx of the affected digit.
i. What are the differential diagnoses?
ii. What diagnostic procedures will establish a definitive diagnosis?
iii. Assuming this is a bacterial osteomyelitis, what is the appropriate treatment and associated prognosis?
iv. Assuming this is a neoplasm, how would treatment and prognosis be different?

97b

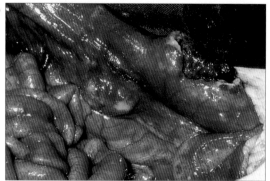

97 i. The usually sharp outline of the abdominal organs is hazy and blurred because of fluid accumulation in the abdominal cavity. The most likely diagnosis is peritonitis. Free gas may be seen if there is gastrointestinal perforation (97b).
ii. Most cases of septic peritonitis are diagnosed accurately by cytologic examination of fluid obtained by paracentesis or lavage. Intra-abdominal injury or disease was accurately detected by needle paracentesis in 47% and by lavage in 95% of cases in a clinical evaluation of 129 dogs and cats.
iii. Incomplete abdominal closure (open abdominal drainage). A mortality rate of 48% has been reported. Other techniques of peritoneal drainage are less successful in draining the abdominal cavity.

98 The four devices are:
• Elizabethan collar or plastic restraint collar (the collars must be big enough to prevent reaching peripheral body parts such as feet and tail, or inhibit neck flexion).
• Body brace or side bars for animals that will not tolerate a collar (aluminum rods secured to the side of the body to inhibit neck and body flexion).
• Hobbles to prevent animals from scratching.
• A wire muzzle (will protect from self-trauma and allows the animal to drink).

99 i. Bacterial or fungal osteomyelitis, squamous cell carcinoma, malignant melanoma, apocrine gland (sweat) adenocarcinoma, severe paronychia and dermatofibrosis associated with renal adenocarcinoma in German Shepherd Dogs.
ii. Biopsy of the digit and culture (bacterial and fungal) of tissue samples. Histologic analysis should include special stains to identify a potential infectious etiology. In this case, excisional biopsy or amputation of the digit is preferred since it is also the initial phase of therapy for all differential diagnoses being considered. In endemic areas fungal titers (e.g. coccidioidomycoses, histoplasmosis, etc.) are performed. Concurrent fine-needle aspirate or cutting needle biopsy of the popliteal lymph node is indicated.
iii. Excision of affected tissues and a short course of postoperative antibiotics (based on culture and sensitivity results). The bone changes present in phalanx III are so severe that resolution of clinical signs is unlikely without amputation. The prognosis is excellent for complete resolution.
iv. Digit amputation is the initial therapy. Lymph node biopsy and thoracic radiographs are performed to stage the tumor. The most common tumor types at this site are squamous cell carcinoma, malignant melanoma and sweat gland adenocarcinoma. All three of these tumors have a propensity to metastasize to the regional lymph node and lungs. Because of this expected behavior pattern, adjuvant chemotherapy or radiation are often implemented for best results. Small tumors limited to the local area have a better prognosis. The short-term prognosis is fair but long-term prognosis is often poor, especially for squamous cell carcinoma and malignant melanoma of the nail bed.

100 The facial view of a 16-week old Boston Terrier is shown (100a).
i. What is the diagnosis?
ii. What are the principles of surgical repair?
iii. What problems may occur postoperatively, and what is the prognosis for successful surgical correction?

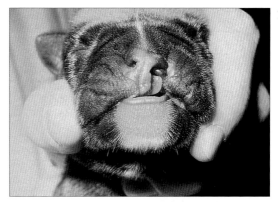

100a

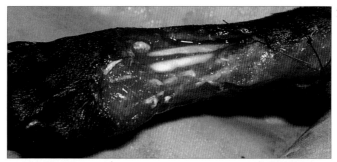

101a

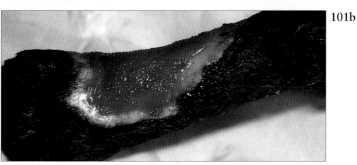

101b

101 This open wound (101a) in a young mixed-breed dog was sustained in an automobile accident. Extensor tendons are exposed. No fractures are present.
i. What is the immediate plan for this wound and what is the long-term goal?
    The open wound is shown three weeks after treatment (101b). All tendons are covered by healthy granulation tissue and a zone of epithelialization is seen surrounding the granulation tissue.
ii. What is done now?

100b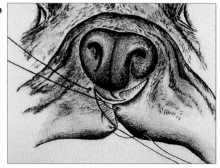

100 i. Primary cleft palate or 'harelip'.
ii. Closure of the floor of the nasal orifice, modified Z-plasty for cutaneous closure, the medial cleft margin is used to reconstruct the philtrum area, adequate flap size for good vascularity and low tension on the suture line. The dorsal suture advancing the laterally created flap medially to the bed of the medially created rotation flap is shown (**100b**). The ventral suture rotates the medial flap ventrolaterally to the ventral aspect of the lateral advancement flap bed.

iii. Postoperative problems include wound dehiscence from excess tension or licking of sutures. If the size of the dehiscence is 3 mm or less, healing by second intention is usually adequate. If dehiscence disrupts the repair, a period of 2–3 weeks is allowed for healing and decreased inflammation before further surgery. Generally, the prognosis is good for successful repair and acceptable cosmesis.

101c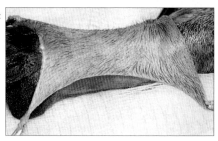

101d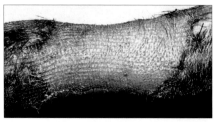

101 i. The wound is cleaned and debrided. Because of considerable tissue loss, primary closure or delayed primary closure cannot be considered. The wound is treated open, allowing it to contract and epithelialize, and making further decisions weekly as the wound heals. Contracture deformities must be avoided and large areas of new thin epithelium are not able to withstand daily normal trauma. A reconstructive procedure is done without delay if one or both of these conditions start to occur.

ii. After three weeks there is a clean, healthy wound. It becomes apparent that further contraction will affect the digits, and further epithelialization will produce a large area of thin, delicate epithelium on the front of the paw (**101b**). The simplest and quickest way to cover this wound is by free skin graft. A large single sheet of full thickness or thick split thickness skin is used because strong skin with good hair growth is desired. This is an excellent wound for grafting. The surface is flat, smooth and well vascularized. A rim of epithelium and one millimeter of the surface granulation tissue is removed. The graft is obtained from the lateral body wall and draped over the wound with hair follicles pointing ventrally (**101c**). The graft is sutured loosely so that it overlaps the skin at the margins of the wound. The graft is bandaged with a non-stick primary layer bandage. The graft is shown at three days when 100% take is expected (**101d**). Full thickness grafts survive, have good hair growth and do well when a favorable body part is selected for the graft. Thin split thickness grafts also take well; however, they tend to be dry and devoid of hair.

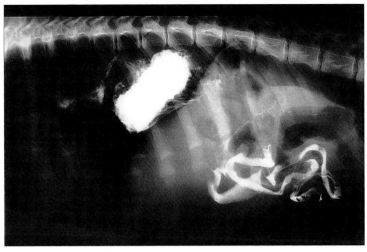

102

102 An eight-month-old, male English Bulldog is presented with a history of hypersalivation and regurgitation. On physical examination, mild dyspnea is noted. A contrast esophogram is performed and a lateral view radiograph is shown (102).
i. What is the diagnosis and what are the different types or categorizations of this abnormality?
ii. What is the surgical treatment for this problem?
iii. What is the prognosis?

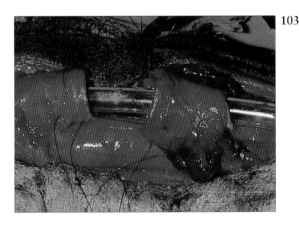

103

103 A cervical tracheal laceration caused by a dog fight in a two-year-old, castrated male Dachshund is shown (103). The endotracheal tube is introduced through a temporary tracheostomy and the laceration is distal to the tracheostomy. The laceration involves approximately three tracheal segments.
i. What are the expected presenting clinical signs?
ii. After confirming the diagnosis what steps are taken to stabilize the patient?
iii. Describe your approach to treatment (include suture patterns and suture type).
iv. What complications might occur?

102 i. Hiatal hernia. These hernias are classified as congenital or acquired (in animals most are congenital), and as a type I sliding hernia or type II periesophageal hernia (in animals most are type I). With type I hernias the phrenicoesophageal ligament is stretched, allowing the gastroesophageal junction to herniate back and forth into the thorax. With type II hernias the gastroesophageal junction remains stationery and the gastric fundus herniates through the esophageal hiatus alongside the esophagus.
ii. This condition is rare in animals and the best surgical approach remains controversial. Successful treatment of three animals with hiatal hernia using a combination of three surgical techniques has been described. A modified Nissen fundoplication is performed to reduce gastroesophageal reflux, in conjunction with suture reduction of the esophageal hiatus and placement of a left fundic tube-gastropexy. The gastrostomy tube provides the additional advantages of allowing nutritional support, bypass of the esophagus and surgery site, and facilitates decompression of the stomach in the early postoperative period. Gas distension, presumably from an inability to belch, can cause discomfort after surgery.
iii. The prognosis for complete relief of clinical signs is guarded. A review of reported cases shows approximately 25% success, and a mortality rate of 64%.

103 i. Expected clinical signs include dyspnea, subcutaneous emphysema, air transgression through the open wound and pneumomediastinum.
ii. Tracheal laceration and respiratory distress is treated as an emergency. Stabilizing measures include intubation or tracheostomy to provide a patent airway, and oxygenation. The cuffed end of the tube must pass beyond the site of the laceration.
iii. Perioperative antibiotics are administered and a ventral midline approach to the cervical trachea is performed. Surrounding tissues are assessed and debrided as necessary. Recurrent laryngeal nerves are identified during exploration.

The affected tracheal cartilage and mucosa is debrided and realigned. Approximately 50% of the trachea can (in theory) be resected in adult animals before stenosis and dehiscence (due to tension) become a major concern. Sutures are limited to the number necessary to reappose the trachea without excessive tension. A simple interrupted suture pattern which penetrates the cartilage of tracheal rings adjacent to the laceration is best. The suture material should be non-absorbable and monofilament with the knots on the external surfaces.

Other techniques include encircling tracheal ring sutures rather than penetrating sutures, suturing of the annular soft tissue, and techniques such as fibrin glue or argon laser welding. To relieve tension, encircling sutures may be placed two to three rings away from the primary wound. In larger dogs, steel sutures with Teflon stents can be placed through the tracheal rings in a horizontal mattress pattern. The site is lavaged and surrounding soft tissues sutured over the anastomosis to provide a seal and eliminate dead space. If dead space or wound contamination is excessive, a Penrose drain is placed.
iv. Potential complications include infection or abscess formation, dehiscence and stricture. All animals with injuries to the cervical region are assessed for laryngeal paralysis. This patient had bilateral laryngeal paralysis which required arytenoid lateralization two weeks after tracheal anastomosis.

104 A nine-year-old, male Golden Retriever has abdominal enlargement, a palpable central abdominal mass and gross hematuria. Abdominal radiographs show only one normal kidney and a large mass. You suspect a kidney tumor.
i. What is the diagnostic imaging test of choice to confirm your clinical suspicion?
ii. What type of renal tumors are most frequent?
iii. What is the surgical technique of choice for renal tumor excision?

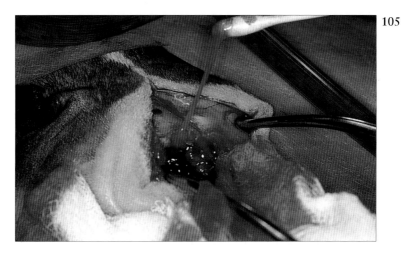

105

105 A seven-year-old, male domestic shorthair cat is presented for chronic bilateral mucopurulent nasal discharge. There is no concurrent facial deformity or epiphora. On oral examination, moderately severe dental tartar formation and pyorrhea is seen.
i. What are several possible causes for the nasal discharge?
ii. What tests will help determine the diagnosis?
   The frontal sinus exposed at surgery is shown (**105**); the cotton applicator shows the viscosity of the discharge present.
iii. What are two surgical treatments for this animal assuming the diagnosis is chronic sinusitis?

104 i. Ultrasonography is probably the most informative and cost effective imaging technique to be combined with survey radiographs for suspected renal tumors. Ultrasonography allows investigation of both kidneys, para-aortic lymph nodes, liver and vena cava for signs of tumor involvement. Excretory urography is an alternative if ultrasonography is unavailable. Computed tomography or magnetic resonance imaging is also extremely useful to evaluate local and regional tumor involvement.

ii. Canine primary renal tumors affect older males more than females and 90% are malignant. Tubular adenocarcinomas are most frequent, and are often bilateral. Metastases are present in >50% of cases (lymph nodes, lungs, liver, bones) at the time of diagnosis. Tumors can also be of mesenchymal (20%, e.g. fibrosarcoma) or embryonal (10%, e.g. nephroblastoma) origin. Lymphoma is the most common renal tumor in cats.

iii. Unilateral renal cancer is best treated by complete ureteronephrectomy, and retroperitoneal muscle resection if capsular extension has occurred. The renal vein is ligated early in the dissection process to minimize the potential for metastases. Partial nephrectomy is sometimes used for surgery of bilateral renal tumors in which a benign histologic diagnosis is made. Survival times >10 months are reported for 20–30% of dogs with renal tumors treated by surgery alone. Death is usually from metastasis. Renal lymphoma is best treated with chemotherapy.

105 i. Chronic sinusitis, bacterial rhinitis (usually secondary to mycotic infection or neoplasia), foreign body, tooth abscess, oronasal fistula and cleft palate. Important characteristics that often indicate etiology include pattern and type of discharge, whether discharge is unilateral or bilateral, and the presence of facial deformity or epiphora.

ii. Open-mouth ventrodorsal (or intraoral dorsoventral) and rostrocaudal skyline radiographs of the skull are made in addition to standard views. Changes such as turbinate destruction and airway opacities are often subtle. Perfect positioning and exposure are mandatory, therefore anesthesia is required. Computed tomography or magnetic resonance imaging is also useful if available.

Copious retrograde nasal flush is performed using a Foley catheter placed in the nasopharynx. All discharged material is carefully examined for foreign matter.

Rhinoscopy is used to inspect for foreign material and neoplastic or fungal lesions, and to gather cytology and histology samples.

Nasal biopsy is performed by curette, endoscopic biopsy instrument, or taking a core biopsy blindly with the plastic sleeve of an i/v catheter or large urinary catheter.

iii. Lavage and surgical drainage into the nasal cavity or sinus obliteration. The sinus is trephined with an intramedullary pin and a small diameter tube is placed percutaneously into the hole, through the sinus, and out to the nasal cavity to establish drainage. If the sinonasal aperture is blocked or narrowed, the sinus is opened and the aperture widened.

Obliteration is indicated if drainage cannot be established or sinus disease recurs. The frontal sinuses and caudal nasal cavity are exposed. The mucosal lining is debrided away (preferably with a power burr), the sinus is packed with fat graft and the wound is closed over a drain.

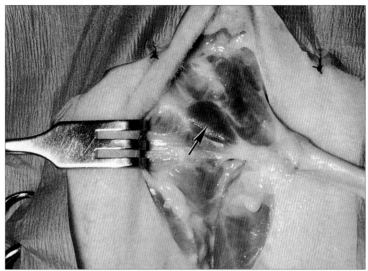

106 A four-year-old, castrated male Siamese cat was presented for a third episode of urethral obstruction. A Wilson and Harrison perineal urethrostomy was performed (106).
i. Assuming the cat is clinically stable, what radiographic procedure may be indicated before surgery is performed?
ii. Describe two methods of transecting the ischiocavernosus muscle (ICM) (arrow in 106) to avoid excessive intraoperative hemorrhage.
iii. What are potential postoperative complications and their predisposing factors?
iv. What are suitable suture materials for urethral suturing?

107 An eight-year-old, spayed female Poodle is treated for necrotizing pancreatitis by partial pancreatectomy.
i. What, if any, special considerations are made for postoperative nutritional support?
ii. Whether you decide this animal needs special nutritional support or not, what type of diet will you choose to feed after surgery, and when will you begin feeding?

108 i. What are two important variables for autoclave sterilization, and what are the minimum values for effectiveness?
ii. Why is steam added to the system?
iii. List two methods of monitoring sterilization, and advantages and disadvantages of each.

106 i. A positive contrast urethrogram is used to rule out another site of urinary obstruction if one is suspected clinically.
ii. Elevation of the ICM from its origin on the ischium; ligation of each ICM and transection near its insertion on the ischium.
iii. Rough dissection predisposes to urinary incontinence if branches of the pudendal nerve are damaged. Failure to incise the penile urethra to the level of the bulbourethral glands, incomplete release of tension on the urethra from inadequate transection of the ICMs (arrow in 106) or ventral ligament of the penis, self-mutilation to the urethra postoperatively and use of an indwelling catheter predispose to urethral stricture. Excess hemorrhage occurs if the ICM is transected in the muscle belly, if there is inadequate ligation of the corpus cavernosum penis after penile amputation, and if the urethra is not incised on the dorsal midline.
iv. Small gauge (4-0), synthetic, monofilament non-absorbable sutures on a swaged on taper-cut needle are preferred. Absorbable sutures are not recommended because absorption of these sutures when exposed to air causes an inflammatory reaction and possible granuloma formation.

107 i. Anorexia and vomiting are likely postoperative sequelae to this case. Because of disease severity and the magnitude of the surgery, energy requirements for this animal will be high. Nutritional support after surgery is needed to maintain an anabolic state. Because vomiting is likely to occur and the gut aboral to the pancreas is functional, placement of a jejunostomy feeding tube is indicated. Adequate nutrient intake cannot likely be maintained with oral, esophageal or gastric feedings.
ii. Diet type is chosen based on: special nutritional needs of animal, route of feeding, and convenience factors (i.e. cost, availability, palatability, etc). This animal has moderate to marked metabolic stress and is subject to glucose intolerance. Calories should be mostly derived from protein and fat. Because of poor pancreatic function fat sources should be less in quantity and highly digestible. Postoperative gastrointestinal ileus predisposes to small intestinal bacterial overgrowth; fructooligosaccharide supplement will help reduce pathogen overgrowth. Because a jejunostomy tube is chosen for feeding, a liquid isosmotic diet is selected. Maldigestion is probably present to a degree, so a monomeric diet is a better selection than polymeric diet.

108 i. Time and temperature. Higher temperatures require less time for sterilization. Recommended settings are 120°C for 13 minutes. Five to ten minutes are sufficient to destroy most microbes and 3–8 minutes are recommended as a safety margin. Unwrapped instruments may be autoclaved at 131°C for three minutes.
ii. Steam is more effective than dry heat for sterilizing materials. Steam must directly contact surfaces of microbes. Heat is transferred to the organism and water condenses, resulting in protein denaturation and microbe destruction. Dry heat destroys microbes by oxidation and requires more time and higher temperatures.
iii. Chemical indicators (autoclave tape or indicator strips) undergo color change at a specific temperature. They are easily used and are inexpensive, but they provide no indication of time at a given temperature. Chemical indicators are best used as a sign that a pack has completed an autoclave cycle, not that it is sterile. Biologic indicators use the temperature resistant spore of *Bacillus stearothermophilus*. After autoclaving, the indicator is cultured and assessed for signs of growth. This is most accurate and reliable, but is more time consuming and expensive.

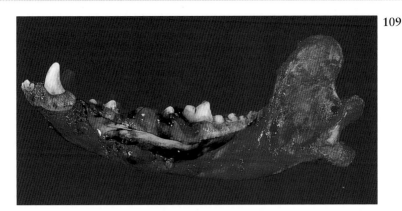

109

109 The hemimandible from a ten-year-old dog that presented with a mass in the oral cavity and a foul odor in the mouth is shown (109).
i. List the three most common malignant canine oral tumors.
ii. Which of these tumors carries the most favorable long-term prognosis for survival and which has the worst?
iii. This particular tumor was histologically diagnosed as a fibrosarcoma. What is the treatment?

110 This dog (110) was pre-sented for persistent licking of the penis and redness of the tip of the penis.
i. Name the condition pictured.
ii. Which breeds are most com-monly affected?
iii. How does the condition occur?
iv. How would you treat the condition?

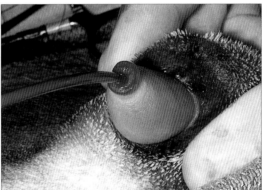

110

111 A large wound was created by resection of a soft tissue sarcoma. Primary closure will result in tension on the wound margins. List three suture patterns that alleviate tension and the advantages and disadvantages of each.

109 i. Malignant melanoma, squamous cell carcinoma and fibrosarcoma (in order of prevalence). In the cat, squamous cell carcinoma and fibrosarcoma are the most prevalent.
ii. Squamous cell carcinoma has the best long-term prognosis in dogs. Local invasiveness of this tumor is limited and the incidence of distant metastasis is low. Malignant melanoma has the poorest long-term prognosis. Although local control can be effectively achieved in approximately 90% of cases, the incidence of metastasis to the lungs and regional lymph nodes is 80–90%. Median survival time is 7–8 months (25% alive at one year) from the time of diagnosis.
iii. Fibrosarcoma has a highly invasive growth pattern and a low propensity for distant metastasis (approximately 20%). Complete resection can be difficult, especially when the tumor is on the lingual side of the mandible or crosses midline on the maxilla. With aggressive resection local control is achieved in approximately 55% of cases. Median survival time is 7–8 months (40% alive at 1 year). Neoadjuvant radiation can be used to shrink tumors before surgery, and adjuvant radiation used to treat incomplete resection margins. Oral fibrosarcomas generally have limited response to chemotherapy. The best way to improve treatment success is to diagnose this tumor-type early and treat it aggressively.

110 i. Urethral prolapse.
ii. The condition occurs almost exclusively in the English Bulldog.
iii. Urethral prolapse can occur following irritation from genitourinary tract infection or excessive sexual stimulation.
iv. Treatment is directed toward elimination of underlying infection and surgical management of the prolapse. Initial therapy involves reduction of the prolapse using a lubricated catheter, and placement of a purse-string suture. The suture is tied tightly enough to prevent recurrence but not tight enough to result in obstruction. The suture is removed in five days. If prolapse recurs, or if there is necrosis and drying of the mucosa initially, amputation of the affected mucosa is indicated. Excision is performed by incising the penile and urethral mucosa for half the circumference of the penis. The urethral mucosa is sutured to the penile mucosa with simple interrupted sutures of fine (e.g. 4-0) absorbable material. Once half of the prolapse is incised and sutured, the remaining urethra is excised and sutured in a similar manner. Incising half of the circumference initially prevents retraction of the urethral mucosa and eliminates the need for stay sutures.

111 Horizontal mattress sutures placed at a distance back from the wound and over a stent will relieve tension on the primary suture line. The disadvantages of this suture are that it may cut through tissue (this is less likely with a stent) and it reduces circulation at the wound edge.

Vertical mattress sutures placed at a distance back from the wound margins will also relieve tension on the suture line. Vertical mattress sutures allow increased circulation to the wound edge as compared to horizontal mattress sutures, and they should be placed over a stent to prevent tissue tearing.

Far-near, near-far sutures approximate the wound margin and relieve tension with less compromise to circulation than horizontal mattress sutures and less tendency to tear tissue than either mattress pattern.

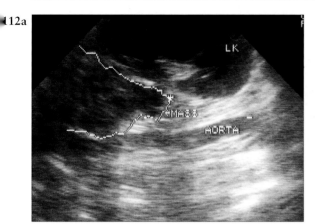

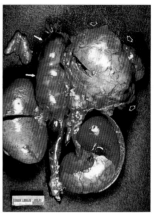

112 A 15-year-old, spayed female Cocker Spaniel underwent abdominal ultrasonography (112a) to evaluate a mass that was detected on abdominal radiographs located in the area of the left kidney and adrenal gland. Ultrasonography revealed a large adrenal mass cranial to the left kidney closely associated with the aorta. A necropsy specimen of an adrenal mass (open arrows) invading the caudal vena cava (thrombus delineated by white arrows) in another patient is illustrated (112b). Both patients had exhibited signs of restlessness and weight loss, and were diagnosed with hypertension.

i. What is the most likely kind of adrenal tumor in both these patients?
ii. Aggregates of extra-adrenal chromaffin cells usually are located near sympathetic ganglia. When tumors of chromaffin cells occur in these extra-adrenal sites, what are they also known as?
iii. Signs associated with adrenal medullary tumors are vague in animals and often go unnoticed, explaining why many of these tumors are diagnosed on postmortem examination. Clinical signs are due to the tumors' ability to produce and secrete excess catecholamines. These signs can be persistent but are usually paroxysmal, complicating diagnosis. Other symptoms reported are related to the invasive nature of some of these tumors. What clinical signs or related conditions are associated with this tumor?
iv. What pharmacological agents can be used to lessen the effects of excess catecholamine release in patients with pheochromocytomas in order to prepare them for surgery or for medical management of the symptoms?

113 An owner calls to tell you that three days after you performed ovariohysterectomy on her six-month-old Dalmatian, the incision split open and intestines were dragged through the grass. The owner sensibly grabbed the dog and wrapped the intestines and abdomen in a clean towel. She is calling on her car phone to tell you that she is coming to your clinic.
i. What is your initial treatment of this dog?
ii. What factors other than too much exercise might lead to dehiscence?
iii. How will you close the abdominal wound this time?
iv. Are antibiotics indicated, and if so, what will you administer?

112, 113: Answers

112 i. Pheochromocytoma.
ii. Paragangliomas or extra-adrenal pheochromocytomas.
iii. Episodic release of excessive amounts of catecholamines can induce hypertension, congestive heart failure, cardiac arrhythmias, restlessness, weakness, polyuria, polydipsia and muscle tremors. Invasion into the adjacent vena cava can result in venous obstruction posterior to the tumor leading to abdominal distension, ascites and hind-limb edema.
iv. Pharmacologic agents used for treatment of excess catecholamine secretions are alpha- and beta-adrenergic blocking agents. *Phenoxybenzamine*, a long-acting alpha-adrenergic blocker, is the preferred drug because it is given orally and is effective. *Prazosin*, a selective alpha-1 antagonist, is not a good choice due to its short duration of action. *Phentolamine*, another alpha-adrenergic antagonist, can be given i/v and is useful in the perioperative period to control hypertension. *Propranolol*, a beta-blocking agent, is useful in emergency control of tachycardia. However, to avoid a severe hypotensive episode due to unopposed alpha-adrenergic vasoconstriction of peripheral vessels, the use of a beta-blocker must be preceded by an alpha-blocker.

113 i. Prepare the following supplies: sterile drapes, surgical gloves, warm crystalloid lavage solution, a sterile bowl, sterilized surgical supplies and an i/v catheter. The dog is anesthetized and the towel is unwrapped. Wearing sterile gloves, the intestines are placed on a sterile drape, copiously lavaged to remove gross contamination, replaced in the abdomen, and the abdominal wall rapidly closed with a continuous suture. The skin is aseptically prepared and the dog taken to surgery for thorough cleaning of the intestines and wound repair.
ii. Since dehiscence happened after only three days, wound healing abnormalities are unlikely in this case. Potential surgical technique errors include: too small a suture size, too much space between interrupted sutures, using chromic gut in a continuous pattern in the abdominal wall, placing fewer than 5–7 throws at the ends of a continuous suture line, handling the suture with needle holders, and incorrectly placed sutures in the linea alba. Removal of sutures by the animal might also have contributed to dehiscence.
iii. Abdominal wall layers are difficult to recognize even three days after surgery. Subcutaneous tissues are adhered to the external rectus fascia and must be dissected free. Rather than trying to recognize the linea alba or external rectus fascia, it is easier to place wide sutures that incorporate the entire abdominal wall. Since the field is potentially contaminated, monofilament suture, either absorbable or non-absorbable, is recommended. For a 20–25 kg dog, at least size 2-0 suture material is used. Simple interrupted sutures, placed 1 cm apart, reduce the chance of suture breakage should the dog continue to be overly active. The subcutaneous tissue and skin are closed routinely, and an Elizabethan collar is used.
iv. A broad-spectrum antibiotic such as cephalexin (20 mg/kg p/o tid) is indicated due to the risk of peritonitis developing.

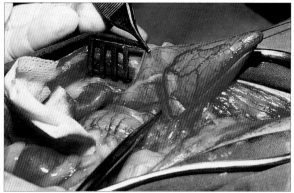

114

114 In the dog in 91, the ureter can be visualized extramurally as it courses along the lateral side of the bladder (114).
i. List the different treatment options for this case, and for other morphologic types of ureteral ectopia.
ii. As far as continence is concerned, what prognosis is expected after treatment of ectopic ureter? What are the causes and treatment options for postoperative incontinence?
iii. What are the major complications of ureteral ectopia surgery and how are they avoided?

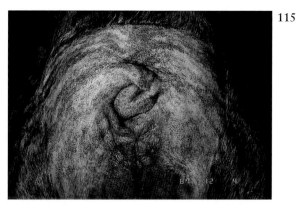

115

115 The tail and perineum of a two-year-old, female English Bulldog is shown (115). The owners report a one year history of odor and moist discharge from the area. Previous evaluation by another veterinarian diagnosed anal sacculitis. The dog was treated with cephalexin and topical antibiotic ointments, and the owners reported a good response initially. More recently, medical management has had limited success.
i. What are several differential diagnoses?
ii. Physical examination reveals deep furrows in the skin around the tail filled with a purulent discharge. A pelvic radiograph of the dog shows deformity of the coccygeal vertebrae. What is the definitive diagnosis?
iii. What are the medical options for treatment of this problem, and what are the shortcomings?
iv. What are the surgical options for this problem?

114 i. If severe unilateral hydroureter and hydronephrosis are present, ureteronephrectomy is considered.

Ureteroneocystostomy is used for extramural ectopic ureter. The ureter is reimplanted into the trigone after its distal extremity has been severed. Microsurgical technique is often necessary for the cat because of the small ureteral lumen.

To treat intramural ectopic ureter, ventral cystotomy is performed. A normal ureteral opening is seen on one side of the trigone and a submucosal ridge caused by the ureter coursing under the mucosal surface is seen on the other. The bladder mucosa and ureteral wall are incised longitudinally. The mucosal edges of the bladder and ureter are apposed using 4-0 to 7-0 absorbable material (monofilament is preferred). The distal portion of the ureter is occluded by passing sutures around it from the serosal surface of the bladder wall.

Surgical correction of ureteral trough is by excision of a strip mucosa from each side of the trough and then closure with a simple continuous pattern of 4-0 absorbable material.

ii. Surgical treatment of intramural ectopic ureters has a better prognosis than extramural ureters. Studies report that about 50% of animals remain incontinent after surgery. Urethral incompetence, reduced bladder capacity and failure to ligate the distal ureter adequately are possible causes. Urethral pressure profile and cystometrogram are recommended prior to surgery, especially in Siberian Huskies. Phenylpropanolamine therapy (alpha agonist) can eliminate or significantly reduce sphincter incompetence in about 50% of cases.

iii. Stomal stenosis can occur causing hydroureter and hydronephrosis. Good surgical technique using magnification and small size sutures helps prevent this complication. If transplantation is done close to the bladder neck, an indwelling catheter can be used as a stent for 4–6 days until inflammation and edema has subsided. Concurrent urinary tract infection is common and should be treated adequately based on culture and sensitivity.

115 i. Anal sacculitis, perianal fistulae, tail fold pyoderma, vulvar fold pyoderma.

ii. Tail fold pyoderma secondary to deformity of the coccygeal vertebrae. This abnormality is known colloquially as a 'corkscrew tail'.

iii. Tail fold pyoderma can be treated medically like any other pyoderma: broad-spectrum systemic antibiotics (first generation cephalosporin, amoxicillin-clavulanic acid or trimethoprim-sulfa) and topical wound care by clipping the hair, cleansing the skin folds with an antibacterial shampoo and application of a topical antibiotic ointment and drying solution. The difficulty is this therapy does not treat the primary problem, and rapid recurrence of signs is common after discontinuing medications. Medical management is useful before surgery to reduce infection and the often copious inflammatory discharge.

iv. Surgical treatment for tail fold pyoderma includes resection of the skin folds, with or without tail amputation. Most surgeons perform concurrent tail amputation because without it the problem often fails to resolve. An elliptical incision is made around the affected area and the tail folds are resected en-bloc with the coccygeal vertebrae. Drains are placed as needed to vent dead space that can not be closed by suturing.

116 This is an oral view of a ten-year-old Labrador Retriever with a smooth well delineated mass on the premaxilla (**116**). The owners first noted the mass approximately six months earlier and they report it has grown in size about 50% since then.
i. What are the differential diagnoses for this lesion?
ii. What diagnostic tests would you perform?
iii. What treatment do you recommend?

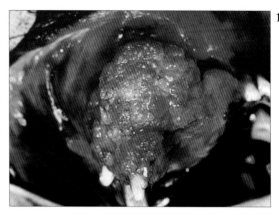

116

117 A 10-year-old, male German Shepherd Dog is presented for acute collapse. The owner reports mild weight loss, and increased lethargy over last month. Abnormalities noted on physical examination are pale mucous membranes and weak pulses. The abdomen seems distended and tender on palpation.
i. What diagnosis do you suspect?
ii. What further diagnostic tests are indicated?
iii. Surgery is performed and the diagnosis is splenic hemangiosarcoma. What is the prognosis?

118a   **118b**

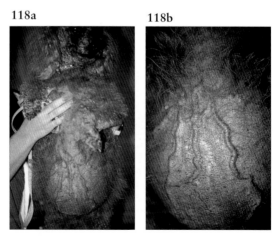

118 This 12-year-old, spayed female Poodle (**118a**) presented with a history of weakness, lethargy and exercise intolerance of two years duration. The owner's current concern is the abdominal distension. You notice the engorged state of the epigastric veins (**118b**) and recommend abdominal ultrasound. The sonogram demonstrates a right adrenal tumor which appears to be invading the caudal vena cava.
i. What is the most likely diagnosis?
ii. What clinical findings would support this diagnosis?
iii. What laboratory test would confirm the diagnosis?
iv. Explain the ascites and venous congestion.

116 i. Epulis, tumor of dental origin, fibrosarcoma and osteosarcoma. These tumors tend to have a smooth mucosal surface and are often well delineated. Rostral position and a slow growth history are most typical of an epulis. Epulides are classified as acanthomatous, ossifying and fibromatous epulis. All are benign but tend to be locally invasive.
ii. Intraoral radiographs are used to determine bone margins needed for resection. If a diagnosis of malignancy would alter the owner's desire to treat the animal, an incisional biopsy is performed. If malignancy is diagnosed, the tumor is staged according to the TNM system.
iii. Rostral maxillectomy is the treatment of choice for this lesion regardless of histologic diagnosis, because local tumor control can very likely be provided with little surgical morbidity. The diagnosis was acanthomatous epulis (the most invasive form of epulis), and requires wide resection for complete removal. Tumors of dental origin and epulides have an excellent prognosis (100% local control) following complete resection. Epulides can also be successfully treated by radiotherapy; however, there is a small chance for delayed secondary malignancy at the irradiated site. Be aware that histologically, acanthomatous epulis can be confused with squamous cell carcinoma and vice versa. If there is doubt about the histologic diagnosis, the pathologist should be consulted.

117 i. Hemoabdomen and secondary hypovolemia from a ruptured splenic hemangiosarcoma, hemangioma or hematoma.
ii. Abdominal radiographs are helpful to confirm peritoneal effusion, splenomegaly or hepatomegaly. Thoracic radiographs are made to rule out pulmonary metastases. A hemogram may reveal regenerative anemia if hemorrhage has been chronic, thrombocytopenia, or the presence of schistocytes or other fragmented red blood cells. The most helpful diagnostic test is four-quadrant abdominocentesis; recovery of fresh blood is an indication for surgery.
iii. The long-term prognosis for ruptured splenic hemangiosarcoma is considered poor; median survival after splenectomy is less than three months. Surgery followed by adjuvant chemotherapy provides a median survival of 3–6 months. The combination of vincristine, doxorubicin and cyclophosphamide (VAC) appears to be the most effective. In a recent study, median survival time was approximately 190 days using the VAC protocol after surgical cytoreduction.

118 i. Pheochromocytoma is most likely but adrenal adenocarcinoma cannot be ruled out without further investigation.
ii. Clinical laboratory data are often normal, although hypercholesterolemia is common. Most dogs with pheochromocytoma are hypertensive (blood pressure elevations 164–325 mmHg systolic, and 110–198 mmHg diastolic), and other causes in dogs are few. Pheochromocytoma should be suspected in animals with hypertension, anxiety and hypercholesterolemia.
iii. Dogs with pheochromocytoma may have high levels of circulating catecholamines. Because of difficulties evaluating blood catecholamine concentrations, urine catecholamines and their metabolites are measured for definitive diagnosis. Urine is collected for 24 hours and 15 ml of 6N hydrochloric acid added. Epinephrine, norepinephrine, metanephrine, normetanephrine and vanillylmandelic acid concentrations are determined.
iv. Ascites and congestion of the caudal superficial epigastric veins are most likely from a tumor thrombus occluding the caudal vena cava (see **112b**).

119 With regard to the female Poodle in **118**, describe how you would remove the mass.

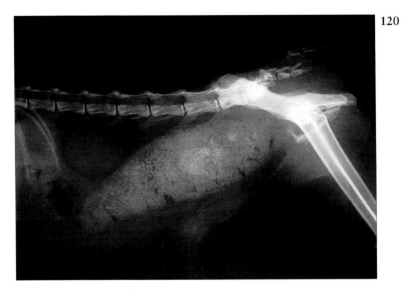

120

120 A five-year-old, domestic shorthair cat was presented with signs of obstipation, anorexia, vomiting and weight loss. A lateral abdominal radiograph of this patient is shown (**120**).
i. What is the diagnosis?
ii. Describe the medical and surgical therapy.
iii. What is the quality of enteric function of cats after surgical treatment for this problem?

121 Name this instrument (**121**) and describe its use.

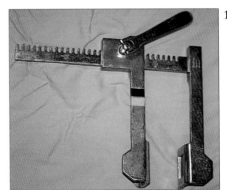

121

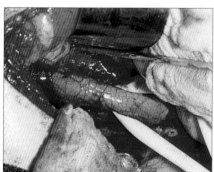
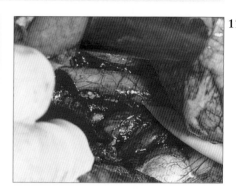

119 If the tumor thrombus within the vena cava is small, a Satinsky clamp is used to isolate the area for venotomy. In this case, the tumor thrombus was large and flow through the vena cava was occluded using Penrose drains (**119a, b**) or Rumel tourniquets placed around the vena cava cranial and caudal to the tumor. With these tourniquets compressed, flow through the cava is suspended allowing venotomy and tumor removal. In order to re-establish flow through the vena cava quickly, a Satinsky clamp is applied across the venotomy after tumor removal. The tourniquets are then released and circulation re-established. With the Satinsky in place, the venotomy is closed routinely.

120 i. Acquired (idiopathic) megacolon.
ii. Medical therapy provides only temporary relief, but should be utilized first and until it is no longer effective. Acute episodes of constipation are treated with laxatives and enemas. Chronic treatment is provided by use of stool softeners, increasing dietary fiber content and treatment with motility modifiers (bisacodyl, cisapride). Surgical treatment is by subtotal colectomy. The ileocecocolic valve can be spared (colorectal anastomosis) reducing bacterial reflux into the small bowel, or it can be excised (ileorectal anastomosis) reducing the likelihood of redistension of the colonic remnant.
iii. In one study no subclinical or clinical evidence of abnormal bowel function was found in normal cats after subtotal colectomy. Bowel movements occurred only slightly more frequently compared with normal cats, and the only significant difference between the two groups was a higher serum cobalamine concentration in the cats in which colectomy was performed.

121 Finochietto rib spreader. It is used during intercostal thoracotomy to spread the ribs. The blades are placed between the ribs and the lever is turned; since there is no quick release mechanism to remove the rib spreader, the lever must be turned counterclockwise until the arms come together. Finochietto rib spreaders are available in various sizes including a child size with 38 × 45 mm blades and a 152 mm spread, and standard sizes with 48 × 65 mm blades and 203 mm, 254 mm and 305 mm spreads. A Finochietto Debakey infant rib spreader is also available with a blade size of 19 × 21 mm and an 85 mm spread.

122 i. What three variables affect sterilization by ethylene oxide?
ii. A red rubber polypropylene and Teflon catheter have just been sterilized with ethylene oxide gas. How long should each item be aerated prior to contacting tissue, and why is aeration necessary?
iii. How can ethylene oxide sterilization be monitored? List two methods and the advantages and disadvantages for each.

123 The proximomedial aspect of the hindlimb of a dog, three weeks after an abrasive, degloving injury, is shown (123).
i. What type of wound healing is occurring?
ii. What are the characteristics of this healing pattern?
iii. How could this wound be treated to enhance wound healing time?

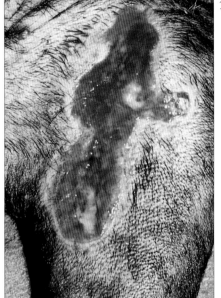
123

124 You are planning to remove a 1.5 cm diameter basal cell tumor located in the flank region of a six-year-old, male Labrador Retriever. The dog will go home with the owner two hours after surgery.
i. What pain control method will you use?
ii. What pain medication will you advise the owner to give the dog, if needed, once the dog is home?

122 i. Concentration, temperature and humidity. Doubling ethylene oxide concentration decreases sterilization time by approximately one-half. Activity of ethylene oxide doubles for every 10°C increase in temperature. Twelve hours should be allowed for room temperature sterilization (25°C) by ethylene oxide, and four hours at a temperature of 55°C. Minimum relative humidity of 33% is essential for ethylene oxide to enter cells, where it causes alkylation of proteins and blocks metabolic reactions.
ii.

	Mechanical aeration	Natural aeration
Red rubber catheter	18 hours	55 hours
Polypropylene tubing	12 hours	48 hours
Teflon catheter	48 hours	168 hours

Aeration is needed because ethylene oxide becomes trapped in rubber and certain plastics and is toxic to mammalian cells. Time is allowed after sterilization for the molecule to diffuse from exposed materials.
iii. Chemical indicators show a color change after exposure to a minimum concentration of ethylene oxide. They do not indicate gas exposure for the required sterilization time, and are best used as a sign of exposure to ethylene oxide, and not a marker of sterilization.
Biologic indicators use spores of *Bacillus subtilis* var *globigii* because this organism is resistant to ethylene oxide. This is the most reliable and accurate indicator, but is expensive and cultures take up to seven days.

123 i. Second intention wound healing. The large, purulent cutaneous defect is allowed to close by granulation, wound contraction and epithelialization without surgical apposition by sutures or staples.
ii. This type of healing is characterized by granulation tissue formation, myofibroblastic contraction producing centripetal movement of the skin, and peripheral re-epithelialization to achieve complete wound coverage. These processes begin after the inflammatory phase, approximately three to five days after wounding.
Drainage is optimal with this type of wound healing, making infections rare. While the time and expense of surgery are avoided, wound management is prolonged by slower healing time. Disfigurement or loss of function from excessive wound contracture should be considered in the decision to manage a wound by second intention healing.
iii. Debridement and lavage of exposed tissues, and surgical closure of the wound (third intention wound healing) by skin graft, skin flap or primary apposition, would shorten healing time. A wound drain is placed if there is concern for continued infection or excess fluid production.

124 i. Regional infiltration of the surgery site with bupivacaine (2–3 mg/kg) before the surgical incision is made will prevent sensitization of the spinal neurons, thus reducing postoperative pain. Additional pain control could be achieved by using oxymorphone (0.05 mg/kg i/v) as a premedicant.
ii. Buffered aspirin (10 mg/kg p/o q 12 hours) can be administered by the owner at home.

125 The dog shown (125) has severed his superficial and deep digital flexor tendons jumping through a plate glass window.
i. What type of suture materials are best suited for repair of the tendon?
ii. Name three suture patterns that are well suited to this repair and the advantages and disadvantages of each.
iii. What postoperative treatment will this dog receive?

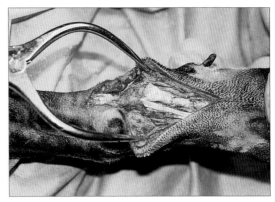

126 This is an oral view of an eight-month-old dog with multiple, proliferative lesions of the labial mucosa (126). The patient was asymptomatic.
i. What is the diagnosis?
ii. What treatment would you perform?

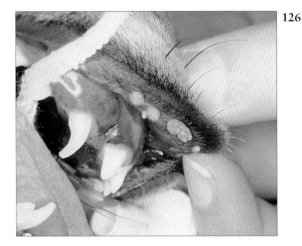

127 Cyanoacrylates are used successfully as a tissue adhesive. Isobutyl-2-cyano-acrylate has been used as a tissue adhesive for closure after feline declaw. Name three desirable properties of this adhesive and one disadvantage. What are some potential complications related to the use of tissue adhesives for feline declaws?

125 i. Monofilament non-absorbable suture. Monofilament suture is preferred because of decreased tissue drag and less destruction of the tendon's intrinsic blood supply. Non-absorbable suture is used because tendon healing is often prolonged (>5 weeks). Polypropylene or nylon are preferred for their minimal tissue reaction; stainless steel is susceptible to cyclic loading and failure, or cutting through tissues.
ii. The Bunnel–Meyer suture pattern has excellent strength and resists suture pull out, but it decreases intrinsic blood supply to the tendon resulting in prolonged wound healing. The Modified Kessler suture (locking loop suture) has equal strength to the Bunnel–Meyer without disruption of the intrinsic blood supply, and decreases tendon gap formation at the anastomotic site. The three-loop pulley suture pattern has greater strength than the locking loop suture and effectively prevented gap formation in one study. The disadvantage of this suture is that a large amount of suture material is exposed and may contribute to adhesion formation.
iii. In humans, early passive motion enhances tendon healing. In animals, we cannot limit activity to passive motion. The anastomosis is protected by external coaptation (Robert Jones bandage or cast) for three to four weeks, after which limited weight bearing is begun. By five weeks, the tendon has approximately 56% of its initial strength. This is well above the 25–33% strength needed for walking activity, but is not sufficient for activities such as running or jumping.

126 i. Oral papillomatosis.
ii. These lesions resolve spontaneously and no specific treatment is necessary. However, confirmation of the disease is appropriate and may help assure particularly concerned clients. A small dissection scissor may be used to 'snip' off one of the lesions, which is submitted for histopathologic assessment.

127 Desirable properties of tissue adhesives include a long shelf life; can be stored at room temperature; good handling properties such as the ability to be spread easily to a thin film; rapid polymerization in the presence of moisture; no pressure required to achieve a short cure time; and the ability to produce a flexible yet strong bond. Most adhesives are non-toxic and non-antigenic, and they can be sterilized in ethylene oxide.

The major disadvantage is slow biodegradation. In experimental studies, moderate amounts of adhesive could be detected in the dermis for several months after application.

Potential complications of tissue adhesives include wound infection, fistulation, dehiscence, tissue toxicity, granuloma formation and delayed healing. These complications are more likely to occur if the tissue is ischemic, contaminated, infected or otherwise compromised. If tissue is compromised to the point that it will not heal with sutures, it will not heal with tissue adhesives. Discomfort to the pet may result from the presence of foreign material in a wound located on weight-bearing surfaces such as feline declaw wounds. Lameness had been reported after adhesive use for feline declaw.

128 A four-year-old, cryptorchid male dog is presented with a history of vomiting, lethargy and pain in the lumbosacral region. On abdominal palpation, a firm, painful caudal abdominal mass was identified. There was no evidence of pain elsewhere and the remainder of the examination, including rectal examination, was normal. Abdominal radiographs revealed a soft tissue mass in the caudal abdomen. Sonography showed a hypoechoic mass was present cranial to the bladder. The kidneys and prostate were normal.
i. What are the differential diagnoses for this dog?
ii. What additional diagnostic tests are indicated?
iii. What is the most probable diagnosis?
iv. What is the treatment for this condition, and what is the prognosis?

129 The postoperative view of a surgical procedure performed on the ear of a dog is shown (129).
i. Name the surgical procedure.
ii. Describe the procedure. Be sure to include anatomic landmarks that are used when performing this surgery to ensure that it is done correctly.
iii. List indications for this surgery (be specific).

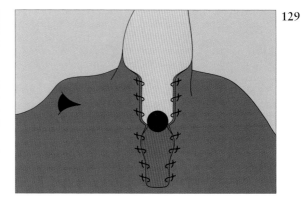
129

130 A 12-month-old, male Poodle was presented for recurrent *E. coli* urinary tract infections.
i. What differential diagnoses are considered, and what diagnostic plan would you propose?

As part of the evaluation an excretory urogram was performed (130).
ii. What is the radiographic diagnosis?
iii. Describe the surgical and/or medical management of the abnormality seen (130).

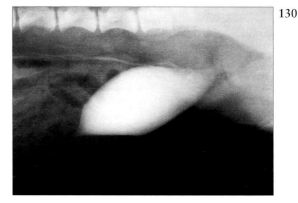
130

105

128 i. Differential diagnoses include testicular neoplasia, testicular torsion, gastrointestinal neoplasia and infected periprostatic cyst.

ii. Hemogram and serum chemistry profile to evaluate for signs of concurrent systemic disease (e.g. anemia, uremia, hypoproteinemia). Urinalysis is indicated to identify urinary tract infection and neoplasia and to assess urine concentrating ability. Radiographs can be used to identify organ of origin, but ultrasound is most useful to identify the mass and differentiate parenchymal consistency.

iii. Testicular torsion is most likely in this case because of the presence of pain, cryptorchidism, and the animal's young age. Radiograph and sonogram results also support this diagnosis.

iv. Treatment is exploratory laporatomy and orchidectomy. Testicular torsion occurs primarily in young to middle-aged cryptorchid male dogs and neoplasia is frequently associated with torsion (6/13 dogs in one report). The prognosis is good for full recovery in the absence of testicular neoplasia with metastasis or anemia (secondary bone marrow suppression warrants a guarded prognosis).

129 i. Lateral ear canal resection (modified Zepp procedure).

ii. Important landmarks include the tragohelicine incisure (rostral to the tragus) and the intertragic incisure (caudal to the tragus). Incisions are made parallel to one another originating from each of the incisures, continued ventrally for 1.5 times the length of the vertical ear canal, and the skin reflected dorsally. The incisions are carried through the subcutaneous tissue, and the parotid salivary gland is identified and reflected ventrally if necessary. The blade of the scissors is placed into the vertical ear canal and two parallel cuts (again originating from the incisures) are made through the cartilage extending to the horizontal ear canal. The lateral wall of the vertical canal is reflected ventrally and approximately 1–2 cm is left attached to the base to form a drain board (the remainder is excised). The drainboard is sutured to the adjacent skin in a simple interrupted pattern making sure to penetrate the cartilage.

iii. Indications include removal of inflammatory polyps in the external ear canal, mild chronic otitis externa limitedly responsive to medical therapy or where owners have difficulty medicating the ear, and for thickening of the external ear canal that does not involve or obstruct the horizontal ear canal. Contraindications are chronic otitis externa where the horizontal ear canal is obstructed or calcified, or as the sole treatment for tumors/polyps of the middle ear.

130 i. Differential diagnoses include urolithiasis, pyelonephritis, prostatitis, urachal diverticulum and neoplasia. Diagnostic tests of value include urinalysis, excretory urogram, cystogram and ultrasound evaluation of the urinary tract.

ii. Radiographs show a small diverticulum filled with contrast at the apex of the bladder. Congenital vesicourachal diverticulum is a remnant of the embryonic conduit between the bladder and the allantoic sac. The conduit normally closes completely in the newborn. If it remains patent, it is called a persistent urachus and urine is seen dripping from the umbilicus. If it closes partially, a urachal diverticulum is formed as shown (**130**). The diverticulum acts as a blind pouch which harbors bacteria in a sanctuary site isolated from exposure to antibiotics.

iii. Surgical treatment consists of excision of the urachal tube including the bladder apex and umbilicus. Urine culture and sensitivity are performed at the time of surgery, and infection is treated with an appropriate antibiotic.

131 If the patient in **130** was a cat, how would the treatment be different?

132 A German Shepherd Dog is presented with rectal prolapse (**132**).
i. Name the predisposing factors or diseases.
ii. What are the treatment options?

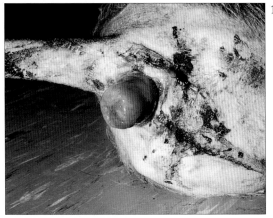

132

133 A nine-year-old Miniature Schnauzer was presented with a four month history of dysuria and hematuria unresponsive to antibiotics. As part of the initial evaluation, survey abdominal radiographs were taken (**133**).
i. Describe how these calculi would be surgically removed.
ii. What postoperative procedure is recommended to ensure successful removal of all the calculi?
iii. Describe the short-term management of this dog.

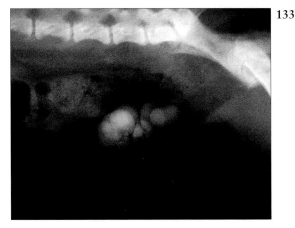

133

134 i. Calculate the ongoing calorie requirements for a 15 kg dog suffering from extensive third degree burns.
ii. What are the protein requirements for this animal, and how would they be changed if the dog had concurrent protein losing glomerulopathy or hepatic insufficiency?

131 In cats, diverticula are frequently detected only after urethral obstruction. Diverticula often regress after resolution of the urinary obstruction, so surgery is not always necessary. Cats are re-evaluated radiographically and by urinalysis four weeks after relief of obstruction to determine if the diverticulum is persistent and surgery is necessary.

132 i. Predisposing factors or diseases include cystitis, dystocia, prostatomegaly, perineal hernia, colitis, rectal foreign bodies, proctitis, rectal or anal tumors, urolithiasis, parasites and postoperative tenesmus.
ii. If the rectal tissue is viable, the prolapse is cleaned and reduced, and a purse-string retention suture of non-absorbable material is left in place for 3–5 days. Alternatively, colopexy can be performed via routine caudal midline laparotomy. Colopexy is best used for recurrent prolapse after removal of an anal purse-string suture, or for chronic intermittent recurrence. Rectal amputation and anastomosis is used when the viability of the rectal tissue is questionable.

133 i. The bladder is isolated from the abdomen with laparotomy pads. Retention sutures are placed at the apex of the bladder and at each side of the cystotomy incision. Calculi are removed, and the bladder and urethra are flushed with saline to dislodge any remaining calculi. Ventral cystotomy affords better visualization of the trigone and ureteral openings, and easier access to the urethra than does a dorsal cystotomy. There is no greater risk of leakage or adhesion compared to a dorsal cystotomy. The cystotomy is closed in one layer with 3-0 or 4-0 synthetic absorbable suture. Suture material should not penetrate into the lumen of the bladder.
ii. Immediate postoperative radiographs are done to detect any calculi remaining in the urinary tract. In studies, up to 15% of dogs and 20% of cats had calculi remaining in the urinary tract after surgery.
iii. Immediate postoperative management requires the bladder be kept empty for several days; the patient must be allowed to urinate frequently, be catheterized or have a closed indwelling urinary collection system placed. Urine is submitted for culture and sensitivity, and the calculi submitted for mineral analysis. Prophylactic antibiotics are continued until urine culture results are returned.

134 i. The resting energy requirement is calculated by using the equation: body weight $(kg)^{0.75} \times 70 = kcal/day$, i.e. in this case: $15^{0.75} \times 70 = 534$ kcal/day. This is multiplied by a disease factor of 1.28 for burn injury; so for this case 684 kcal/day are required. If the intended diet contains 1.2 kcal/g, then 684 kcals ÷ 1.2 kcal/g, i.e. 570 g of food, needs to be fed per day. An individual animal's requirements can vary, so clinical monitoring is important to refine this 'guideline-value'.
ii. The guideline for protein requirement in the dog is 4 g/100 kcal of metabolizable energy in the chosen diet, and for the cat is 6 g/100 kcal.
For this animal, 4 g/100 kcal × 684 kcal = 27 g of protein are required per day. This value would be increased for animals with ongoing protein loss (6 g/100 kcal for dogs, 8 g/100 kcal for cats) such as glomerulopathy, and decreased for animals with protein intolerance (2 g/100 kcal for dogs, 4 g/100 kcal for cats) such as hepatic insufficiency. If a diet ration designed for animals is being used, the protein requirements are likely to be already balanced in the diet. If a human enteral food product is being used, supplementation with a protein module may be required.

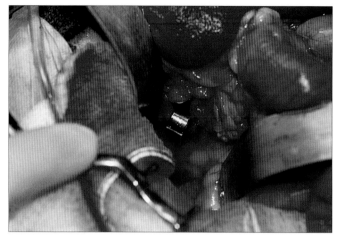

135 A seven-month-old, female Yorkshire Terrier is diagnosed with a single extrahepatic portocaval shunt. Clinical, hematologic and transcolonic nuclear scintigraphy results support the view that the shunt is no longer open.
i. What are the three surgical options available for management of a single extrahepatic portosystemic shunt?
ii. Which of the three techniques described was utilized in this dog (135), and what are the advantages of using this procedure for shunt occlusion?
iii. What are several potential pitfalls with the procedure illustrated above?

136 A four-year-old, spayed female domestic shorthair cat is presented with a history of exercise intolerance and lethargy of several months duration. Thoracic radiographs reveal marked pleural effusion. Thoracocentesis produced the white fluid pictured (136).
i. What is the most likely diagnosis and how can this be verified?
ii. What are four possible etiologies?
iii. What treatment options are available, and what response would you expect?

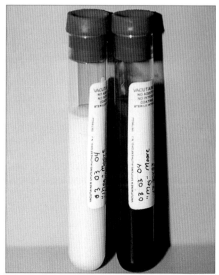

135 i. Complete shunt ligation is ideal but can result in fatal portal hypertension. When the shunt cannot be completely occluded, partial ligation is performed while monitoring portal blood pressure using a monometer and evaluating the splanchnic viscera for signs of congestion. Recently a new tool, an ameroid constrictor ring, has become available to gradually occlude the shunting vessel .
ii. Ameroid constrictor ring. This is a circular metal band with a casein lining and a key mechanism that allows it to be placed around the shunting vessel. The lining of the ring slowly expands, gradually occluding the shunting vessel between 28–35 days after placement. With gradual occlusion portal flow through the liver slowly increases avoiding development of severe portal hypertension. The ameroid constrictor also eliminates a second surgery to occlude completely the shunting vessel as is often done following partial ligation.
iii. Disadvantages to using an ameroid constrictor include increased expense ($40–$60), until familiarity is gained, the ring can be somewhat cumbersome and awkward to place, and depending on the extent of vessel manipulation during placement venous thrombosis may occur. The ameroid ring is in the early stages of clinical application and long-term evaluation of its efficacy is not available.

136 i. Chylothorax or pyothorax. Chylous fluid is a white or pink, opaque fluid that will not clear when centrifuged. The predominant cell type on cytologic analysis is the lymphocyte. An ether clearance test can be used to verify fluid type, although a more objective way is to compare the cholesterol and triglyceride content of pleural fluid and serum. Chylous fluid has a higher triglyceride content than serum and a normal or low cholesterol content. Fluid associated with pyothorax may appear similar but often has a foul odor. Cytologically, neutrophils and bacteria are usually abundant.
ii. Etiologies for chylothorax include: trauma, cranial mediastinal mass, cardiomyopathy, lung lobe torsion and heartworm infection. When no obvious underlying disorder is found, the term idiopathic chylothorax is used.
iii. Treatment depends on etiology; if possible, the inciting cause is eliminated or treated. Medical management is directed at decreasing chyle formation by feeding a fat-free diet and draining the pleural space. Medium chain triglycerides are used as dietary fat supplement since they are absorbed directly into the portal system and not transported in chylomicrons by the lymph system. The pleural space is drained via thoracostomy tube and continuous suction.
    Surgery is indicated in cats that do not have underlying disease and when medical management has failed. Options include thoracic duct ligation, shunting procedures (pleurovenous or pleuroperitoneal) such as the Denver shunt, passive pleuroperitoneal drainage through a diaphragmatic mesh, or pleurodesis. Medical and surgical therapy of this disease can be frustrating. Reported success rates for cats treated with thoracic duct ligation are variable (20–40%). Potential complications of chylothorax include lobe torsion, pleural fibrosis and intrathoracic infections.
    The best approach for treatment is a combination of dietary management to decrease the formation of chyle, and surgical ligation of the thoracic duct combined with passive pleuroperitoneal drainage through a diaphragmatic mesh.

137 A two-year-old, female Pekingese is presented for evaluation of stertorous breathing. The owners report the dyspnea becomes worse when the dog is excited. On oropharyngeal examination, the soft palate extended through the rima glottidus (137).
i. What is the diagnosis?
ii. What is the treatment? Describe the procedure in detail.
iii. What are the potential complications?

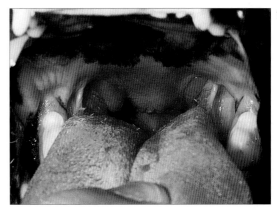

137

138 This is a five-year-old, spayed female, mixed-breed dog that presented for reluctance to eat and the presence of a swelling and draining sinus ventral to the medial canthus of her eye (138).
i. What is the diagnosis and list possible causes for this problem?
ii. List tests helpful to confirm the diagnosis, and what you would expect to find for each result?
ii. Discuss two options for treatment of this problem?

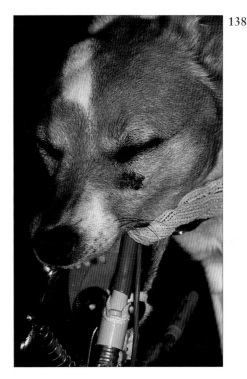

138

137 i. Elongated soft palate. The palate should not interfere with the rima glottidis. Elongated soft palate is often one component of brachycephalic airway syndrome. BAS consists of stenotic nares, elongated soft palate, everted laryngeal saccules and occasionally hypoplastic trachea.

ii. Treatment is by staphylectomy or surgical resection of the obstructing portion of the palate. The soft palate should slightly overlap the epiglottis but not interfere with the rima glottidis. At surgery, stay sutures are placed in the lateral aspects of the soft palate and it is retracted rostrally. The palate is resected using a cut-and-sew technique: excess palate is excised in one-third portions and immediately oversewn with absorbable suture material. Enough palate is resected to prevent interference with the larynx, but should not be resected beyond the caudal aspect of the tonsils (136). If BAS is present, concurrent rhinoplasty, tonsillectomy and laryngeal sacculectomy is performed.

iii. The most common postoperative complication is pharyngeal edema. This is minimized by using gentle technique, avoiding electrocautery, and administering an anti-inflammatory dose of corticosteroids (e.g. dexamethasone 0.1 mg/kg) before surgery. Hemorrhage is best controlled by limited incision and rapid suturing of the mucosal edges; pressure is applied if hemorrhage persists after suturing. Excessive palate removal may cause nasal reflux by failure to cover the nasopharynx during swallowing.

138 i. Carnassial tooth abscess (malar abscess, facial fistula or sinus), although other teeth can be involved. Common causes include slab fractures with pulpal exposure, extension of a deep periodontal pocket, or concussive disease of the root apex.

ii. Oral examination for fistula formation; color of the tooth crown as an indication of viability; palpation of the apex for swelling; and percussion of the root to assess the animal's response. Percussion may confirm extension of infection into the periodontal ligament space as accumulation of fluid in this space increases pressure and produces pain on percussion.

Radiographs are indicated but may not always give the diagnosis; overlying structures can impair evaluation (foraminae and bony trabeculae can mimic endodontic lesions). Common radiographic signs of tooth abscess are changes in the shape and continuity of the lamina dura, and the width and shape of the periodontal ligament, indicating periodontal and pulpal necrosis. In chronic cases an apical osteolytic lesion may be evident. Accurate positioning is imperative, and if there is question about apical lucency, the view is repeated and the contralateral tooth radiographed for comparison.

iii. Treatment of carnassial tooth abscess is by either root canal therapy or extraction. Indications for root canal therapy are: exposure of the pulp cavity from tooth fracture, attrition or caries; facial swelling; intraoral or extraoral fistula; gingival inflammation with pocket formation in a combined periodontal/endodontic lesion; extraction is performed when financial constraints are imposed. Recurrence is possible if a root tip is left in place.

Concurrent antibiotic therapy for anaerobes and Gram-positive aerobic cocci is instituted. Appropriate choices include tinidazole, metronidazole, clindamycin or amoxicillin-clavulanate.

139 This is a rectal polyp in a ten-year-old, male, mixed-breed dog (**139a**).
i. What is the surgical therapy?
ii. What is the prognosis?
iii. What preoperative preparation may be beneficial in this patient?

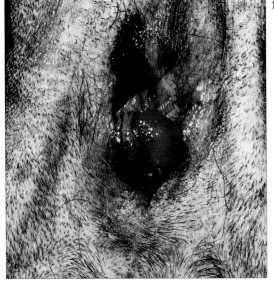

139a

140 The perineum of a nine-year-old, male Doberman Pinscher is shown (**140**). The dog has had a one month duration of tenesmus and soft stools. The owners noted the perineal swelling approximately two weeks earlier, and they report the dog has had no difficulty urinating.
i. What is the diagnosis, and what is the cause of this abnormality?
ii. What are two common surgical techniques for repair of this problem?

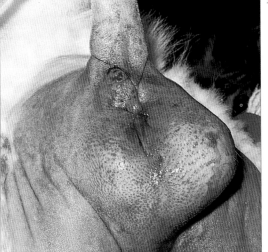

140

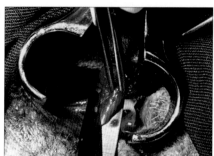
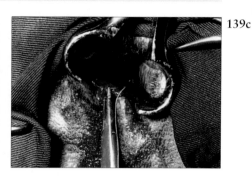

139 i. Small polyps are removed per rectum using electrocautery, surgical excision (139b, c), cryosurgery or simple ligation. Larger polyps or tumors invading the muscularis mucosae may require intestinal resection and anastomosis.

ii. Prognosis is excellent after complete excision, but recurrence can occur with large lesions and new polyps can develop. Concurrent colitis or other source of chronic irritation must be treated. Dogs are periodically rechecked throughout their life to assess for and treat new polyp formation. Malignant transformation occurs in humans and probably dogs, although it has not been proven.

iii. Preoperative preparation is by withholding food for 24 hours and administration of enemas and laxatives. Use of enemas on the day of surgery is not advisable since it increases the risk of contamination from spillage of liquid feces. Preoperative enteric and systemic antibiotics may decrease bacterial contamination of the wound.

140 i. Perineal hernia. Herniation occurs when abdominal contents (fat, prostate, bladder, etc.) rupture through to the perineum, generally between the levator ani and external anal sphincter muscles, from straining against the weakened pelvic diaphragm. Prostatomegaly, colitis or constipation often cause the straining, and a weakened pelvic diaphragm occurs from atrophy (neurogenic, senile, hormonal or metabolic) of muscles forming the barrier.

ii. The 'classic' technique is performed by apposing with preplaced chromic gut sutures (size 0 or 1) the levator ani (coccygeus muscle is used if the levator ani muscle is atrophied), external anal sphincter and internal obturator muscles. The difficulty with this technique is the muscles can be severely atrophied and the sutures are under moderate tension after closure, particularly ventrally, predisposing the herniorrhaphy to dehiscence and failure (up to 45% incidence). The second technique is transposition of the internal obturator muscle. The obturator muscle is elevated from the ischium, transposed dorsally and sutured to the external anal sphincter and levator ani or coccygeus muscles. The advantage is the obturator muscle provides a wider 'patch' for the hernial rent, and consequently sutures are under less tension upon completion. The reported incidence of failure is 5% for this technique. Care is taken to protect the pudendal vessels and nerves which are closely adjacent to the transposed muscle flap. A variation for both techniques is to place lateral sutures in the sacrotuberous ligament rather than the levator ani or coccygeus muscles. The ligament is much stronger than the often atrophied muscles, but greater care must be taken to avoid penetrating the caudal gluteal vessels and sciatic nerve.

141 This is the radiographic image of an eight-year-old, female Poodle presented for evaluation of a distended abdomen and difficulty breathing (141a). On examination, symmetrical alopecia of the flanks, dorsum and perineal region was present. Serosanguinous fluid was collected on abdominocentesis. On sonography of the mid-abdomen the animal had hyperechoic nodular masses caudal to both kidneys. A mass of 4.4 cm diameter with a cystic formation of 2.6 cm diameter is shown (141b).

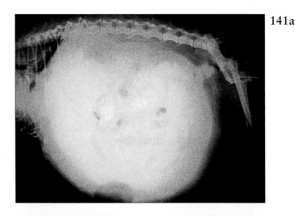

141a

i. Is the radiograph helpful in the diagnosis?
ii. From the information provided on the sonogram, what organ is affected?
iii. What are the most common tumor types for this organ?

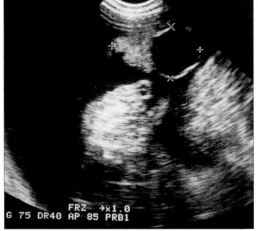

141b

142 Masses removed from the middle ear and horizontal canal of a nine-month-old Siamese cat are shown (142).
i. What is the correct diagnosis, and how is this made?
ii. List four common presenting clinical signs for this condition?
iii. Describe the procedure for removal of these masses, and what is the prognosis for this cat?

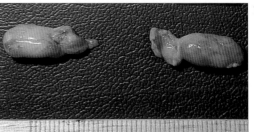

142

141 i. No. The only abnormality seen is a large amount of peritoneal fluid obstructing the view of most of the abdominal organs. It is impossible to determine the origin of the fluid. Ultrasound examination is indicated to study the organs not visible on the radiograph.

ii. The ovary and caudal kidney. This image, combined with the clinical signs, is indicative of a hormone-producing ovarian neoplasia. Cytologic analysis of the peritoneal effusion revealed neoplastic cells.

iii. Ovarian tumors are uncommon in dogs and cats, presumably because animals are so frequently neutered. Epithelial cell tumors such as papillary or cystadenoma/carcinomas are most common (40–50%), followed by sex-cord stromal tumors such as teratoma (30–50%) and germ cell tumors such as granulosa cell tumor (6–20%). Ovarian tumors often cause no clinical signs until they become large enough to create a space-occupying effect. Metastases can affect the lungs, liver, lymph nodes and adjacent kidney. Ovarian carcinoma can cause malignant effusion and intra-abdominal seeding, and frequently affects both ovaries. In general, metastatic rates are low for ovarian tumors (<20%) and complete surgical excision often results in a cure. Once metastases occur the long-term prognosis is poor, although short-term responses have been reported following chemotherapy.

142 i. Bilateral inflammatory polyps (middle ear polyps, nasopharyngeal polyps). Polyps are common in cats and may be congenital. Their presence is confirmed by otoscopic examination of the ear canals, and examination of the oropharyngeal region by retraction of the soft palate rostrally using a spay hook. Radiographs of the pharynx and skull may show the mass, increased opacity of the osseous bullae, thickening of the bullae wall, and sclerosis of the petrous temporal bone. This cat had no evidence of nasopharyngeal polyps.

ii. Aural discharge; a visible mass in the horizontal canal on otoscopy; signs of otitis media or interna; dyspnea or dysphagia if there is extension into the nasopharynx.

iii. Surgical removal of inflammatory polyps is based on polyp location. For nasopharyngeal polyps, an oral approach is used. In the external ear canal a lateral ear resection may be necessary, and those located in the middle ear are excised by ventral bulla osteotomy. These polyps were removed from the horizontal canal following a lateral wall resection, and a ventral bulla osteotomy was performed since the polyps were arising from the middle ear.

For bulla osteotomy the cat is placed in dorsal recumbency with the neck elevated. The bulla is palpated caudal and slightly medial to the vertical ramus of the mandible. A paramedian skin incision is made over the bulla. By separating the digastric muscle from the hyoglossal and styloglossal muscles, the ventral bulla is visualized. The hypoglossal nerve must be avoided. A Steinman pin is inserted into the bulla and the opening enlarged using rongeurs. The cat bulla is divided by a septum that must be opened for complete drainage and curettage. The polyp is excised at its base. Lavage is performed and a drain placed prior to closure. Prognosis is excellent long term, but recurrence is likely if the entire polyp is not removed.

143a

143b

143c

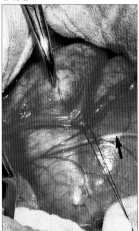 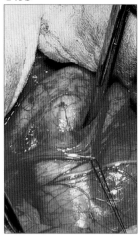 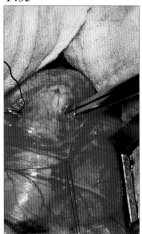

143 These illustrations demonstrate the surgical correction of a cardiac defect (143a–d).
i. Name the condition.
ii. What breeds are predisposed to the development of this condition?
iii. Describe the surgical approach used for this exposure.
iv. What structure is being retracted ventrally with a stay suture, and what structure is identified by the arrow in 143a?
v. Which ligature is tightened first, and what is the Branham reflex?

143d

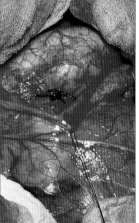

144 Many surgery patients ill from trauma or disease suffer from protein–calorie malnutrition. Nutrient deprivation adversely affects humoral and cell mediated immunity and wound healing, putting animals at increased risk for sepsis and other complications. Nutritional assessment and support is of paramount importance because no patient benefits from starvation.

How do you assess the nutritional status of animals? Discuss history, physical examination, laboratory findings, treatment and disease related factors, and special nutritional status tests.

143 i. Patent ductus arteriosus (PDA).
ii. Miniature Poodles, Pomeranians, Keeshonds, Collies, Shetland Sheepdogs, German Shepherd Dogs, Brittanys and Cocker Spaniels.
iii. A left 4th intercostal lateral thoracotomy. The skin incision is made parallel to the ribs at the caudal border of the scapula. The latissimus dorsi muscle is incised parallel to the skin incision and the intercostal spaces are counted using a hemostat inserted cranially under the latissimus. The insertion of the scalenus muscle is incised leaving enough for the muscle to be reapposed at closure. The serratus ventralis muscle is separated parallel to the direction of the muscle fibers. The intercostal muscles are incised in the middle to avoid damaging the intercostal vessels and nerve along the caudal margin of each rib. Once the pleura is incised, ventilation is assisted. The opening is extended dorsally to the tubercle of the rib and ventrally to the internal thoracic artery which is visualized and avoided. A Finochietto rib spreader is used to maintain exposure. The left cranial lung lobe is packed into the caudal recesses of the surgical field with a moist sponge or laparotomy pad. The PDA is identified between the pulmonary artery and the aorta.
iv. The vagus nerve is being retracted with the stay suture, and the phrenic nerve is identified with the arrow.
v. The aortic side ligature. Once this ligature is tightened, the blood pressure increases and the heart rate decreases – the Branham reflex. After a couple of minutes the size of the pulmonary artery decreases and the ligature on the pulmonary artery side may be tied.

144 Clinicians should gauge nutritional status by assessment of history and diet, physical examination, medical and surgery status and selected clinical chemistries. *History:* owners are questioned about quantity and quality of food intake by the animal (if intake is reduced the duration of decreased intake) and about sources of nutritional loss such as vomiting and diarrhea. *Physical examination:* animals are inspected for loss of lean body mass, poor coat quality, limb edema and pressure sores. Special care is taken in overweight/obese dogs that may still have lost lean body mass. *Laboratory findings:* anemia, lymphocytopenia and hypoalbuminemia are suggestive of protein–calorie malnutrition. Albumin is a poor indicator of actue protein malnutrition because concentrations change slowly; it is more useful for determination of chronic malnutrition. Transferrin, an iron binding and transport protein, reflects acute changes more accurately; low transferrin levels can cause secondary anemia. A lymphocyte count of less than $800/mm^3$ is an indicator of immune suppression and, if due to malnutrition, predominantly involves T-cells. Abnormal values such as these are interpreted with care since disease processes besides malnutrition can result in similar changes. *Treatment and disease related factors:* nutritional intake can be adversely affected by oral and gastrointestinal surgery, chemotherapy and other factors (iatrogenic or disease induced) that cause vomiting, diarrhea or decreased appetite. *Special tests:* in the future, more accurate tests such as calorimetry and nitrogen balance will be used to more accurately and quantitatively assess nutritional status.

145 A German Shepherd Dog is presented for dyschezia and excessive licking of the perianal region (145).
i. What is the diagnosis, and what is the signalment of a typical patient?
ii. Name several treatment options and their approximate success rates.
iii. List the most common potential complication (and its approximate incidence) for each therapy.

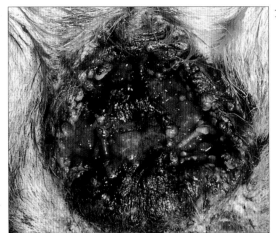

146 This is a view of the labial mucosa in a 12-year-old Labrador Retriever (146). The owner became concerned upon noticing blood-tinged saliva hanging from the left cheek commissure.
i. What is the diagnosis?
ii. What would be considered a palliative surgical procedure for this lesion?
iii. What would be considered a more definitive surgical procedure for this lesion?

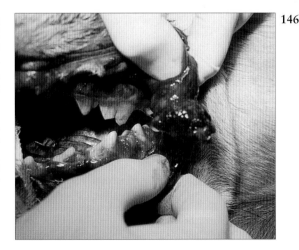

147 Suture material is used in a variety of patterns. There are advantages and disadvantages to each closure pattern. The surgeon should choose a suture pattern that provides optimum security but minimal interference with wound healing.
i. When closing skin, is an inverting or everting suture pattern more desirable?
ii. When closing a wound, what are the advantages and disadvantages of interrupted and continuous suture patterns?

119

145 i. Perianal fistulas. Male, two years of age or older, German Shepherd Dogs or other large breeds are most commonly affected.
ii. Medical treatment can be administered by oral and topical antibiotics, local cleaning and topical antiseptics; results are at best temporary relief of clinical signs. Surgical excision with or without primary closure has a success rate of 60–80%. Cryotherapy or chemical cauterization of the fistulas is successful in 80–90% of reported cases. Deroofing and fulguration has a 60% reported success rate and tail amputation used alone an 80% success rate. Recently, successful treatment had been reported with immunosuppressive drug therapy (steroids, cyclosporin).
iii. The most frequently recognized complications are: surgical excision – recurrence and incontinence (20–60%); cryotherapy – recurrence and stenosis (10–45%); chemical cauterization, deroofing and fulguration, tail amputation – recurrence (20%).

146 i. Malignant melanoma. Benign hyperplasia of pigmented mucosa would be a significantly less likely differential diagnosis.
ii. Submucosal resection of the mass for excisional biopsy will provide short-term resolution; however, tumor recurrence locally, regionally (lymph nodes) or at distant sites (lungs) is likely. The long-term prognosis is poor regardless of treatment for large (>2 cm) melanomas. Small (<2 cm) melanomas often have a good long-term prognosis.
iii. A similar diagnostic work-up as in **19** is recommended for all patients with oral neoplasms. Full-thickness resection of the cheek commissure and a modified neck dissection to remove regional lymph nodes (mandibular, parotid and medial retropharyngeal) is a comprehensive procedure in an attempt to remove as much tumor mass as possible. Cheek reconstruction using a caudal auricular axial pattern flap will provide excellent cosmesis. Follow-up adjunctive chemotherapy may be indicated. This procedure may provide a greater tumor-free interval and improve the prognosis from poor to guarded.

147 i. Skin margins tend to invert as healing proceeds hence suture patterns that create slight eversion are preferable. Simple interrupted, interrupted cruciate and Ford interlocking are all acceptable patterns for dermal closure.
ii. The primary advantage of interrupted patterns is the ability to precisely adjust tension at each point along the wound in accordance with variable spreading forces along its margin. With an interrupted pattern, each suture is a separate entity, and failure of one suture may be inconsequential. The major disadvantage of interrupted patterns is the increased time necessary to tie many individual knots. There is also more foreign material left in the wound when sutures are buried.

The primary advantage of continuous patterns is speed of closure. Less suture material is used and fewer knots are present. This reduces both operative time and the amount of foreign material in the wound. Continuous patterns also form a more watertight or airtight seal. The major disadvantage of continuous patterns is the potential for suture breakage and disruption of the entire line of closure. There is also less precise control of suture tension and wound approximation. The Ford interlocking pattern is a good compromise; it can be applied rapidly, yet provides fairly accurate adjustment of tension at multiple points along the wound.

148 List the steps for proper care of surgical instruments prior to sterilization.

149 The inguinal and cranial thigh regions of a German Short-haired Pointer presented for treatment 48 hours after vehicular trauma are shown (**149**). The dog's vital signs are stable and limb function is unaffected except for the soft tissue wounds.
i. In terms of wound classification based on duration of injury and expected level of contamination, how would this wound be categorized?
ii. What are the treatment options for this case and prognosis for recovery?

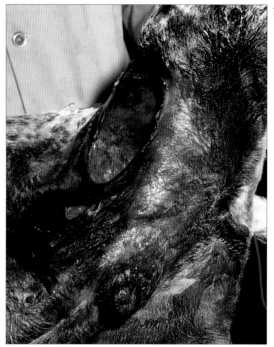

149

150 A nine-year-old, female Doberman Pinscher is presented for ovariohysterectomy. After routine venipuncture your technician notes that the dog continues to bleed. Upon questioning the owner, there is no previous history of surgery other than cosmetic otoplasty and tail docking as a puppy. Delayed hemorrhage at the incision areas was noted at that time by the owner. Examination of the dog is otherwise normal.
i. What is a quick, immediate assessment of this patient's coagulation ability that you can perform in the clinic?
ii. What diagnostic procedures do you wish to perform to further evaluate coagulation status in this dog?
iii. What is the most likely diagnosis, and what presurgical treatment can be used in this patient to temporarily correct the coagulation abnormalities?
iv. What endocrine abnormality can you screen for, which may have important implications for future management of this coagulopathy?

148 Instruments are: (1) rinsed in a weak detergent; (2) cleaned ultrasonically; (3) rinsed in instrument milk; (4) examined to determine working condition. Instruments are first soaked in warm water with a weak detergent to loosen dried blood and debris. Gross contamination is removed before placing the instruments in an ultrasonic cleaner. Ordinary soaps and abrasive compounds are avoided because they leave behind alkaline residues. Ultrasonic cleaning works via cavitation, whereby minute air bubbles are created, expand and implode. This process is more effective at removing tightly adhered soils than other methods of cleaning and is strongly recommended for routine cleaning of instruments. Following rinsing and drying, instruments are quickly rinsed in instrument milk to lubricate moving parts and help prevent corrosion and staining. A final inspection for damage is made when instruments are placed in the pack in an orderly fashion. Sterilization indicators are added for gas or steam sterilization, as appropriate, prior to wrapping.

149 i. An open, contaminated wound of greater than six hours duration, and containing foreign debris and devitalized tissue would be classified as a dirty wound. The reported infection rate for these wounds is 18%.
ii. Treatment for this injury includes: debridement of necrotic tissue; copious wound lavage with sterile saline or antiseptic solution (dilute povidone or chlorhexidine); reduction of dead space; drainage of contaminated tissue pockets; and wound closure. Systemic antibiotics are not required unless signs of systemic disease such as fever, inappetence, toxemia, cellulitis or degenerative leukocytosis are present. Tissue approximation can be by primary or delayed primary wound closure using an adjacent pedicle graft. The prognosis for recovery is fair to good and depends on local and systemic tissue health factors, and the efficacy of surgical treatments.

150 i. The cuticle bleeding time can rapidly determine if a coagulation defect is present. If the cuticle bleeding time is normal (less than six minutes), then significant bleeding during surgery is unlikely; if prolonged, a primary hemostatic defect is present, i.e. vasculopathy, thrombocytopenia or platelet dysfunction.
ii. Examination of a blood smear and platelet count determination. Activated coagulation time (evaluates the ability of whole blood to clot with the contact activator diatomaceous earth). Tests for secondary hemostatic defect or intrinsic clotting system defects: activated partial thromboplastin time (APTT), one-stage prothrombin time (OSPT); fibrin split products (FSP); and factor VIII-related antigen (FVIIIR:Ag) for Von Willebrand's disease (VWD). Bleeding time in this dog was eight minutes, Von Willebrand's factor was significantly decreased and all other coagulation tests were normal.
iii. VWD is associated with prolonged bleeding time, decreased values for Von Willebrand's factor and normal APTT, OSPT and FSP values. Presurgical treatment with either fresh whole blood, fresh plasma (5–10 ml/kg) or fresh frozen plasma (5–10 ml/kg), and desmopressin acetate at a dose of 1 mg/kg s/c will temporarily ameliorate bleeding tendencies. FVIIIR:Ag can be increased in collected blood by pretreating donors with desmopressin acetate.
iv. Hypothyroidism increases bleeding tendencies in VWD patients. Decreased platelet adhesion and prolonged bleeding times have been noted in patients with low thyroid hormone levels alone.

151 With regard to the cat in **96**, you diagnose renal trauma. Is surgery a reasonable consideration and how would you proceed with it?

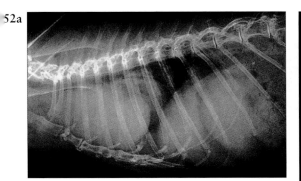

152 These thoracic radiographs (**152a, b**) were made during a routine preoperative work-up on a nine-year-old, spayed female rabbit.
i. What is your radiographic diagnosis?
   A sonogram demonstrated a multilocular, cystic structure in the cranial mediastinum. On cytologic evaluation, a fine-needle aspirate of the mass was highly cellular with the majority of cells being mature lymphocytes.
ii. What is your cytologic diagnosis based on these findings?
iii. What surgical approach would you use to treat this condition?
iv. What major anatomic structures would you encounter and how would you deal with them?
v. What clinical laboratory data are expected to be abnormal with this condition?

153 This is a microsurgical tissue forceps (**153**). It has several features making it suitable for use during microsurgery. Describe these features and their importance for microsurgery.

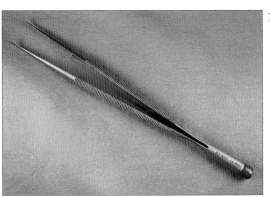

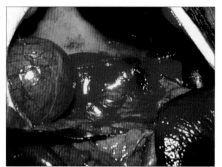

151 If an animal with diagnosed renal/ureteral trauma does not improve with supportive therapy, if severe damage to the kidney is suspected and significant hemorrhage continues, or a urethral tear is diagnosed, exploratory laparotomy is performed. The retroperitoneum is entered via ventral midline laparotomy. In this case, left kidney trauma with secondary hemoretroperitoneum is shown (**151**). Attempts are made to preserve all viable renal tissue and whenever possible partial nephrectomy is performed. Compensatory hypertrophy of remaining glomerulae will occur. The renal artery is occluded with a vascular clamp and partial nephrectomy is performed by excising all terminally damaged renal tissue. Arcuate arteries are ligated and the renal pelvis is sutured closed (4-0 absorbable monofilament). Exposed renal parenchyma is covered by omentum sutured to the capsule. The kidney is replaced and nephropexy performed. For severe trauma ureteronephrectomy is performed. If a ureteral tear or avulsion is present it is primarily repaired, or ureteronephrectomy is performed if injury is severe.

152 i. A cranial mediastinal mass is evident. There is loss of cranial cardiac waist, elevation of the trachea and the cranial lung fields are replaced by the tissue dense mass.
ii. Thymoma.
iii. Median sternotomy is used for removal of a large mediastinal mass.
iv. The internal thoracic artery and vein are avoided along the internal surface of the sternebrae. In large dogs where a saw is used to cut the sternebrae, a flat metal instrument such as a malleable retractor is inserted along the internal surface to protect intrathoracic structures from the saw. Other important structures to identify and avoid include the cranial vena cava and phrenic nerves present along the craniodorsal aspect of the mass. In some cases the tumor surrounds a phrenic nerve and it must be sacrificed. The thymic artery is also found nearby as well and must be ligated to allow removal of the thymoma.
v. Clinical laboratory findings are generally normal. In some patients a mature lymphocytosis ($>20 \times 10^9/l$ ($>20,000/mm^3$)) may be present. Hypercalcemia has been documented in some cases and is suspected to be a result of pseudohyperparathyroidism.

153 The back end of the forceps is weighted so the instrument balances in the groove of the hand created by the thumb and first finger. This allows the surgeon to use the instrument without having to grip it preventing muscle fatigue and tremors. The handles are round which allows the surgeon to roll the instrument between the fingers. During microsurgery, the fingers manipulate the instrument with almost no movement originating from the arms and hands. If the handles are flat, the rolling action performed by the fingers is jerky, while if the handles are round, rolling produces a smooth motion at the tip of the instrument. The tips are miniaturized to allow accurate tissue handling of very fine structures during microsurgery; however, the overall length of the instrument is maintained. Many ophthalmic instruments have an overall short length and must be held between the thumb and first finger. This results in muscle fatigue and tremor.

154 The perianal area of a spayed female Maltese Terrier is shown (154a).
i. Give the diagnosis, and describe the surgical therapy.
ii. Name common postoperative complications.

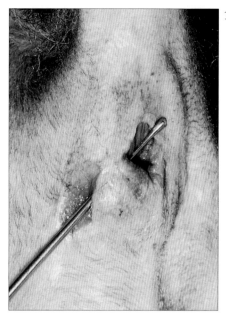

154a

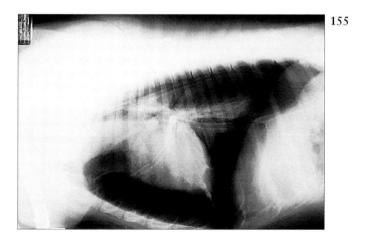

155

155 A six-year-old, male Samoyed presents with a history of an acute onset of dyspnea and cyanosis. Thoracic radiograph is shown (155). There is no history of antecedent trauma.
i. What is the radiographic diagnosis?
ii. What is the suspected disease process and its etiology?
iii. How should this dog be treated, and what is the prognosis?

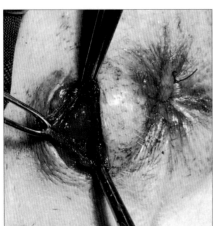

154b

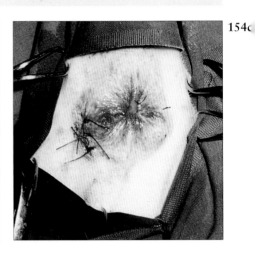

154c

154 i. Ruptured anal sac abscess. Surgical excision is the therapy of choice. Preoperative administration of antibiotics may reduce the inflammatory component and facilitate surgical removal. All anal sac epithelial lining must be removed to prevent recurrences (154b). The wound is flushed thoroughly and may be closed primarily (154c), over a Penrose drain, or left open for healing by secondary intention.
ii. Fecal incontinence, chronic draining tracts, tenesmus, stricture formation and dyschezia.

155 i. Pneumothorax is evident based on elevation of the cardiac silhouette and collapse of the caudal lung lobes. Pneumothorax can be traumatic or spontaneous; in this case spontaneous pneumothorax is most likely.
ii. In a series of 21 dogs with spontaneous pneumothorax, all had underlying pulmonary pathology noted grossly or histopathologically. Bullous emphysema is most common and it is likely that a bleb or bulla associated with this condition ruptured causing pneumothorax.
iii. Although thoracocentesis may be effective in treating traumatic pneumothorax, thoracostomy tube placement is usually necessary for spontaneous pneumothorax. If more than two thoracocenteses are required within 24 hours, tube thoracostomy is performed and continuous suction applied for several days to keep pulmonary and chest wall tissues apposed allowing an adhesion to form. An effective adhesion is often difficult to maintain and recurrence following conservative treatment is high. If pneumothorax persists and there is radiographic evidence of the source, thoracotomy is considered. With bilateral involvement of the pulmonary parenchyma, median sternotomy is performed for partial or complete pulmonary lobectomy to remove diseased tissue.
The prognosis is guarded. Recurrence rates for spontaneous pneumothorax in dogs treated by thoracocentesis or tube thoracostomy is 80% or higher, and with surgery recurrence approaches 25% as other areas of lung can develop bullae which subsequently rupture. Adjunct procedures such as mechanical or chemical pleurodesis may further increase the effectiveness of surgical management.

156 A nine-year-old, male Yorkshire Terrier is presented for a chronic, non-productive cough. The cough occurs primarily when the dog gets excited, and until recently it was manageable with medical therapy. A lateral thoracic radiograph taken during mid-inspiration showed narrowing of the cervical trachea near the thoracic inlet. The radiograph taken at mid-expiration was normal. Screening laboratory work was unremarkable.

i. Why were radiographs taken at mid-inspiration and expiration?
ii. What other diagnostic tests are indicated?
iii. Are there any surgical treatments for this abnormality? Provide details.
iv. What are the success rates and complications of surgical treatment?

157 A ten-year-old, male Collie presented for swelling of the nose (**157a**). The owners noted an intermittent mucopurulent nasal discharge from the left nostril. You suspect a nasal tumor due to the dog's age and presenting clinical signs.

i. List three tumors of the nasal cavity.
ii. A CT scan was performed on the nasal cavity of the dog (**157b**). Describe the findings. Do you still suspect a nasal tumor?
iii. If this tumor is diagnosed as the most common nasal tumor found in the canine, what is the prognosis and list three available treatments?

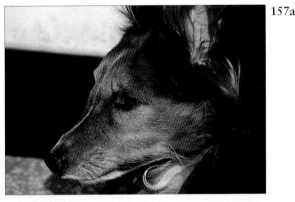

157a

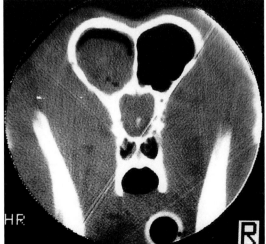

157b

127

156a 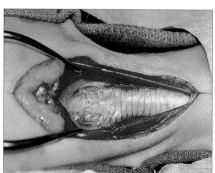 156b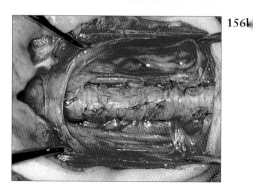

156 i. Tracheal collapse occurs from degeneration and weakening of the cartilaginous tracheal rings (156a). The result is narrowing and dynamic collapse of the large airways (trachea, mainstem and lobar bronchi); the severity and location varies with the phase of respiration. Collapse is more severe in the cervical trachea during inspiration because of the negative intraluminal airway pressure, and in the intrathoracic trachea and lobar bronchi during expiration because of the positive extraluminal airway pressure. The phase specific changes in pressure induce a dynamic collapse that is more apparent radiographically when exposures are made during mid-inspiration and mid-expiration.
ii. Fluoroscopy provides visualization through all phases of respiration and is superior to radiographs. Bronchoscopy is also useful to evaluate the location and severity of collapse, and to allow inspection of laryngeal function and lobar bronchi.
iii. Surgical treatments include chondrotomy, trachealis muscle plication, tracheal resection and anastomosis, and intra- or extraluminal tracheal ring prostheses. Of these, extraluminal polypropylene C-shaped or spiral ring prostheses provide the best results (156b). Prostheses are placed along the collapsed section of trachea (results are poor if there is concurrent lobar bronchi collapse because they cannot be stented) and the wall is sutured to the stent restoring luminal diameter.
iv. Placement of ring prostheses (C-shaped stents) provided elimination or significant improvement of clinical signs in over 60% of treated animals in one report. Animals over six years of age did worse probably due to an increased incidence of underlying disease, such as infection, collapse of the mainstem bronchi and heart disease. Common postoperative complications included persistent cough or dyspnea, and laryngeal paralysis.

157 i. Nasal adenocarcinoma (most common), squamous cell carcinoma, fibrosarcoma, chondrosarcoma, osteosarcoma, lymphosarcoma, hemangiosarcoma and transmissible venereal tumors.
ii. There is a large soft tissue mass in the left nasal passage. There does not appear to be bony lysis nor is there a shift of the nasal septum. Do you still suspect tumor?
iii. If diagnosed as nasal adenocarcinoma, the prognosis is guarded. Eighty per cent of nasal tumors are malignant and are prone to early local invasion and recurrence after therapy. Treatments include radiation (external beam or brachytherapy), photodynamic therapy, cryotherapy, immunotherapy and chemotherapy. Radiation therapy is the best treatment. Mean survival time of dogs treated with surgery and orthovoltage, or cobalt irradiation is 25 months (approximately 60% alive at one year and 40% at two years). Other therapies are considered only palliative.

158 Tumors located in the caudal part of the rectum can be treated surgically by various techniques, depending on the extent of tumor involvement.
i. Name and describe this technique (158a).
ii. Name two alternative approaches that can be used for rectal lesions not involving the anus.
iii. Name the major disadvantages of each technique.

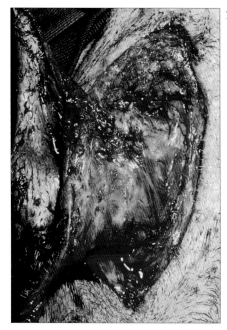

158a

159 A five-year-old, female Boxer is presented for this protruding vulvar mass (159).
i. What are three differential diagnoses for the abnormality shown?
ii. How can these three abnormalities be differentiated?

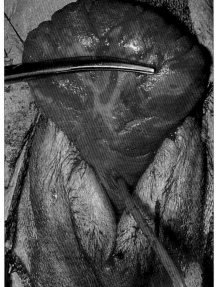

159

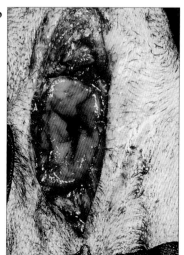
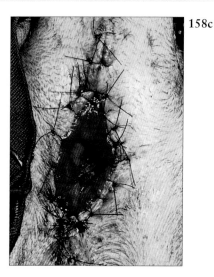

158 i. Rectal pull-through procedure. An incision is made in the skin surrounding the anus or anocutaneous junction, depending on the extent of the tumor. Blunt dissection and caudal traction are performed along the adventitial surface of the rectum. The abnormal part of the rectum is amputated (**158b**) and the rectal end is sutured to the skin (**158c**).

ii. The ventral approach using pubic symphysectomy or pubic osteotomy to gain access to the pelvic canal, or the dorsal perineal approach.

iii. Rectal pull-through: postoperative complications include incontinence, stricture formation and dehiscence. Ventral approach: complicated access to the rectum and postoperative morbidity associated with the osteotomy technique. Dorsal perineal approach: limited access and extensive dissection.

159 i. Vaginal hyperplasia (vaginal edema), vaginal prolapse and neoplasia.

ii. Diagnosis is based on signalment, history of estrus, vaginal examination and urinary catheterization. Vaginal neoplasms occur in older (median age 10–11 years) intact nulliparous females, and are not necessarily related to estrus. Masses are often firm and pedunculated; leiomyoma and fibroma are most common and can arise from any surface of the vagina. Vaginal hyperplasia and prolapse usually occur during the follicular phase of estrus and are associated with physiologic (or pathologic) elevations of estrogen. Hyperplasia is usually seen at the first heat cycle and commonly recurs; prolapse can occur at any age and is most often associated with straining. Vaginal hyperplasia occurs from marked thickening of the vaginal floor cranial to the urethral papilla. The indurated tissue protrudes from the vagina, appearing as a red fleshy mass. The urethra does not become exteriorized and can be readily catheterized by reflecting the mass dorsally and visualizing the papilla. Vaginal prolapse presents as a doughnut-shaped mass from eversion of the complete vaginal circumference. The urethral papilla is commonly exteriorized and is catheterized by visualizing the papilla in the center of the 'doughnut'.

160 With regard to the Boxer in 159, how does the treatment differ for the three diagnostic considerations?

161 The abdominal radio-graph of an 11-year-old, female, mixed-breed dog presented for evaluation of pollakiuria is shown (161a). The patient was previously diagnosed with a 'fibroma' in the neck of the uterus and the owner elected no treatment at that time. On clinical examination the dog had a visibly distended abdomen and on palpation a large firm mass was occupying the mid and caudal abdomen. There was no vaginal discharge, hematuria or hematochezia. Rectal examination was normal. On screening laboratory evaluation only a mild leukopenia and eosinophilia were present.

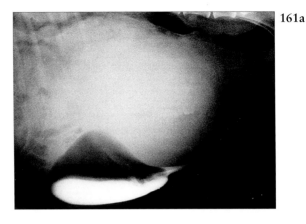

161a

i. What other diagnostic or staging tests are indicated?
ii. What is the treatment and likely prognosis?

162 A deglove injury on the hindlimb of a three-year-old, mixed-breed dog is shown (162). The lateral collateral ligaments of the hock have been avulsed, the interior of the joint is exposed, and several small bone fractures are present. There is 360° of skin loss from below the stifle to the digits.
i. This is obviously a serious wound. What problems and solutions are discussed with the owner?
ii. How can this wound be managed?

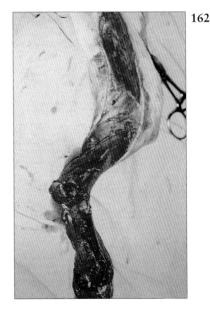

162

160 Treatment of vaginal hyperplasia is by surgical excision of redundant vaginal tissue; without concurrent ovariohysterectomy recurrence is likely at parturition or the next estrus cycle. It is not usually necessary to treat mild vaginal prolapse as spontaneous regression will occur in diestrus. For more severe cases where the prolapsed tissues are suffering from exposure or strangulation, the tissues are reduced using a well lubricated obturator such as a syringe case (episiotomy may facilitate this), a urinary catheter is placed and the vulvar labia are temporarily closed with sutures. If the prolapsed tissues are devitalized, then circumferential resection is performed. Ovariohysterectomy induces permanent regression of vaginal prolapse. Surgery is the treatment of choice for vaginal tumors except transmissible venereal tumor (TVT). Excision generally cures the most common vaginal tumors; TVTs can be cured with chemotherapy.

161b

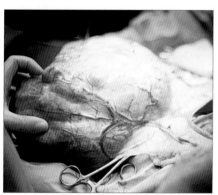

161 i. The presence of a large mass occupying practically the whole abdomen and preventing visualization of other organs is best evaluated by sonography. Ultrasound allows determination of the affected organ, the nature of parenchymal consistency, and is useful to obtain guided needle aspirate or biopsy samples. If this diagnostic tool is not available at a primary care or referral facility, exploratory laparotomy for direct observation, biopsy sample collection or surgical resection is the next best choice. In this case a uterine mass was confirmed by ultrasound examination. There was no evidence of abdominal metastases. Three-view thoracic radiographs (ventrodorsal view and both right and left lateral views) were evaluated for metastases and none were seen. ii. Treatment for uterine neoplasia is ovariohysterectomy (161b). In dogs most uterine tumors are benign (55–90% leiomyomas) and cause no signs. Complete resection is generally curative. Leimyosarcoma was diagnosed in this case. This uncommon tumor type (10% incidence) is more prone to local invasion into adjacent organs, and distant metastasis to the lymph nodes, liver and lungs. With complete resection and no evidence of metastasis, the prognosis is good for tumor control.

162 i. There is no quick treatment of such a wound. The owner must understand the complexity, length and cost of management. Treatment will require 30–50 days and the hock joint will likely be stiff, however it should be possible to salvage the leg.
ii. A clean, healthy, granulating wound surface is first produced to cover all joints, tendons and bones. The wound is cleaned, debrided, and covered by a non-occlusive dressing as a primary layer. The limb is bandaged with an absorptive secondary layer and an external splint is incorporated. With proper care a healthy wound is obtained in about 25 days (see 163).

163 With regard to the injury on the hindlimb of the dog in 162, the wound is shown after 25 days of treatment (163a).
i. What alternatives are considered for definitive care of this wound?
ii. Describe in detail the chosen method.

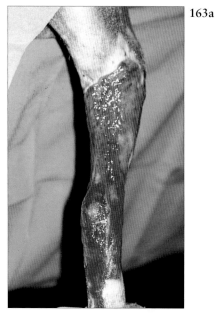

163a

164 This is a ventral view of a five-year-old, mixed-breed dog with a ventral cervical mass (164). The mass, which had been enlarging during a six week period, was fluctuant and non-painful. A cervical mucocele is suspected.
i. What is the simplest diagnostic test?
ii. How would the affected side be determined?

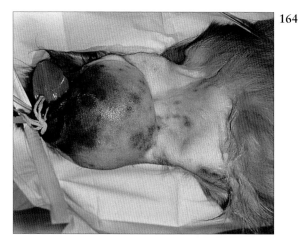

164

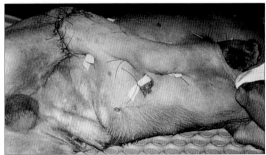

163b

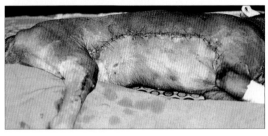

163c

163 i. No loose available skin is adjacent to the wound. Healing by contraction and epithelialization, or undermining and mobilization of skin edges is ruled out. Free autogenous skin grafts can be used; however, a large wound in an area difficult to bandage can require multiple grafts, and the healed area is usually a mixture of skin and epithelialized scar tissue easily damaged by normal trauma. Axial pattern flaps are not useful for this large 360° distal wound. Free microvascular transplantation of a flap requires a suitable artery and vein at the recipient site and special expertise and equipment. A method used successfully and recommended by this author (D.E. Johnston) for large distal open wounds on forelimbs and hindlimbs is a direct bipedicle flap from the lateral body wall.

ii. The leg is placed against the abdominal wall in the conscious animal to determine that the joints have adequate flexibility and that the animal does not resent the maneuver. The skin is marked where incisions are made for entry and exit of the leg. Tissue is excised from the edge and surface of the granulating wound and hemostasis obtained. The leg is inserted beneath the undermined skin through the two incisions, and the abdominal skin is sutured to the leg (**163b**). The leg is then fixed (here an insufficient amount of the paw was available for fixation by a bandage, so the leg was fixed to a body bandage by nylon sutures inserted into the pads). The bandage is changed in seven days and the leg detached in 14 days (**163c**). Sufficiently large flaps are measured and removed to wrap around the medial aspect of the leg by fashioning a wound template before the leg is placed under the body wall skin. This method is technically simple and results in full thickness skin replacement in 14 days. No muscular or neural problems have been seen by this author in six reported cases and no dog that required this procedure has been ruled ineligible because of temperament.

164 i. Fine-needle percutaneous aspiration. Aspiration is useful to diagnose a mucocele (stringy, sometimes blood-tinged fluid with low cell numbers), and to rule-out infectious or inflammatory lesions.

ii. Mucoceles often lateralize when the patient is placed in dorsal recumbency. If the affected side is still equivocal, historical reference to when the mucocele was smaller or sialography may provide information as to the affected side. Sialography can be difficult and time consuming to perform; it is challenging to find and cannulate the sublingual and/or mandibular salivary duct.

165 With regard to the dog in 164:
i. What is the surgical treatment of choice?
ii. Can mucoceles be life-threatening?

166 A two-year-old, castrated male cat was presented for anuria and azotemia after a cat fight. There was marked swelling of the perineal tissues and groin area. A cystogram and urethrogram were performed as part of the evaluation (166).
i. What are three surgical options for treatment of this injury?
ii. The most common complication of urethral trauma is stricture. Which treatment option would have the least chance of causing urethral stricture? Which would have the most?
iii. Describe the after-care of this patient?

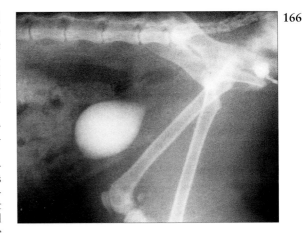

166

167 A 12-year-old, intact male Yorkshire Terrier is presented with signs of tenesmus.
i. The perianal area is shown (167a). Give the most likely diagnosis and list some differential diagnoses.
ii. This tumor is hormone dependent. What hormone is involved, and what disease has been reported to cause this tumor in spayed female dogs?
iii. List three different therapies for this disease.

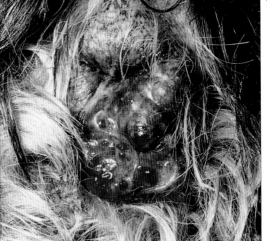

167a

165 i. Resection of the mandibular and sublingual gland/duct complex to a point near the lingual nerve. Mucoceles secondary to saliva leakage from a gland/duct defect rostral to the lingual nerve rarely occur. If the defect is not observed during dissection (often the case) and the affected side was not determined preoperatively, rather than perform more diagnostic tests or wait to see if the mucocele recurs, the opposite mandibular and sublingual gland/duct complex may be concurrently resected. Xerostomia is not a problem following bilateral mandibular and sublingual gland resection as dogs still have bilateral parotid and zygomatic salivary glands.
ii. Yes. Pharyngeal mucocele may cause airway obstruction. This is an emergency situation requiring aspiration of the mucocele and marsupialization. Definitive surgery for this type of mucocele is also resection of the mandibular and sublingual gland/duct complex.

166 i. Primary repair of the urethral rent via pubic osteotomy, with 4-0 to 5-0 synthetic absorbable suture. An intraurethral catheter and closed urinary collection system, or urinary diversion using a Stamey or Foley cystostomy catheter, is indicated for 5–7 days after surgery.
Secondary healing around a soft intraurethral catheter with closed urinary collection system for 7–21 days depending on the size of the laceration and degree of urethral tissue injury. Pubic osteotomy is not necessary in this case.
Prepubic urethrostomy might be required if urethral damage was extensive.
ii. Surgical repair and primary healing over a soft intraurethral catheter would have the least chance, using a catheter alone and allowing secondary healing would have the most chance of causing urethral stricture.
iii. A urinary catheter is maintained for several days to weeks depending on the treatment chosen. In most animals this requires an Elizabethan collar, side brace, or incorporation of the catheter system into a body bandage. The catheter is regularly checked for patency. Urinary tract infections are controlled with use of a closed urinary collection system, and at the time of catheter removal urine is cultured and appropriate antibiotic therapy prescribed.

167b

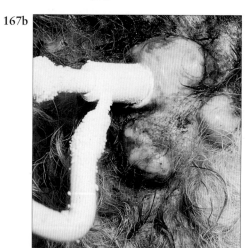

167 i. Perianal gland adenoma. Differential diagnoses include perianal adenocarcinoma, anal sac adenocarcinoma and non-tumorous diseases of the perianal area (anal sac abscess, perianal fistulas, etc.).
ii. Testosterone, pituitary-dependent hyperadrenocorticism.
iii. Surgical resection, cryotherapy (**167b**) and castration. The prognosis for control of perianal adenoma with all three treatments is excellent.

168 A three-year-old, male Labrador Retriever undergoes exploratory laparotomy for intussusception (**168a**). The intussusception was non-reducible and a portion of jejunum was resected.
i. What suture pattern would you use to anastomose the jejunal ends?
ii. What surgical stapling equipment could be used to anastomose the jejunal ends?

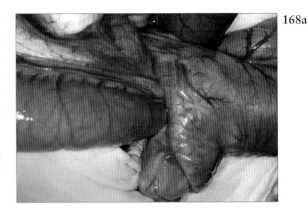
168a

169 A fluid filled mass over the olecranon of a one-year-old, male Great Dane is shown (**169**). The owners first noted the mass two weeks previously and they report it has become approximately 25% larger since that time. It is non-painful.
i. What diagnostic test(s) would be useful to further define this abnormality?
ii. What are two possible treatments for this abnormality, and their significant related complications?
iii. What important management or husbandry change is needed to facilitate treatment and prevent recurrence?

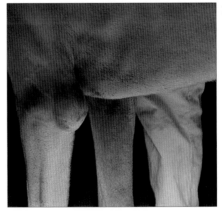
169

170 A four-year-old, female Weimaraner developed this swelling overnight (**170**). The dog has no history of otitis and does not scratch her ears. The owner reports the the dog is kept in a fenced-in yard and enjoys running up and down the fence-line with the neighbor's dogs.
i. What is the diagnosis?
ii. List three potential causes for this condition.

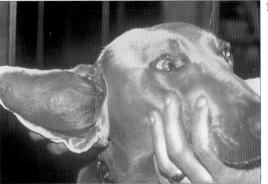
170

168c

168b 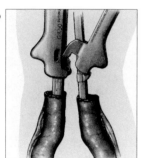 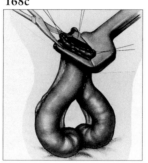 168d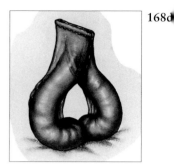

168 i. Appositional sutures such as a Gambee, simple interrupted or simple continuous pattern are preferable. The Gambee suture is less susceptible to wicking of bowel contents than simple interrupted. Inverting or everting patterns can be used; however, they can compromise bowel lumen size and increase adhesion formation respectively.
ii. An anastomosis can be created with the GIA and TA 55 stapling instruments (United States Surgical Corporation Norwalk, CT) (168b). The antimesenteric borders of the segments are apposed and the stapler is fired, creating two double-staggered staple lines to join the bowel. Simultaneously, the knife blade cuts between the double staple lines to create a stoma. Sutures are placed to close serosal and mucosal surfaces at the edge of the single opening that has been created. A TA 55 (168c) is applied across the intestinal edges, locked and activated. Excess tissue is trimmed using the cartridge edge as a guide (168d) to complete the anastomosis.

169 i. Sterile preparation of the skin and fine-needle aspiration of the mass to confirm serous fluid and a diagnosis of hygroma. If the fluid is purulent, culture and sensitivity is performed.
ii. Drainage by fine-needle aspiration and placement of a pressure relieving ('donut' padded) bandage for 2–3 weeks, or open drainage by lancing and placement of Penrose drains for 10–14 days, followed by padded bandaging for another 10–14 days. Significant complications of aspiration are iatrogenic bacterial contamination, and hygroma recurrence. Complications for surgical drainage are more extensive fibrosis and a cosmetic blemish over the elbow, and a small but possible chance for recurrence. Aspiration is most useful for smaller acute hygromas, and surgery for larger more chronic ones. Excision is not appropriate since hygromas are not true cysts. They are more akin to seromas, and the best treatment is one that facilitates the tissue layers healing back together.
iii. An important management change is to alter the surface the animal lies on. Hygromas are generally caused by repetitive trauma from kenneling animals on hard surfaces and change to a softer surface such as carpet or grass is important for resolution and to prevent future recurrence.

170 i. Aural hematoma: blood accumulation between the cartilage layers of the pinna from ruptured branches of the great auricular artery on the inside of the auricular cartilage.
ii. Causes include trauma, parasites, otitis, aural foreign body, and ear canal tumors or polyps. This dog's hematoma was due to trauma.

171 With regard to the dog in 170, describe several procedures to correct this problem. Make sure to discuss postoperative management.

172 A one-year-old, male Miniature Poodle was presented for simultaneous urination from the anus and urethra, hematuria and cystitis. A lateral fluoroscopic image of the contrast cystogram and retrogade urethrogram is shown (172). Contrast is shown passing from the urethra at the pelvic brim into the distal rectum (arrowed).
i. What is the diagnosis?
ii. Describe the best surgical approach to the anomaly.
iii. What other surgical procedure is recommended to be done at the same time?
iv. What is the potentially serious consequence if this condition is left untreated?

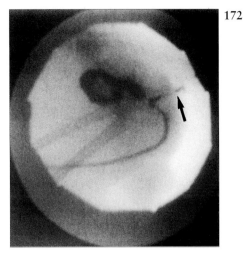

173 An open wound of two years duration in the inguinal area of a five-year-old cat is shown (173). History indicates that the original wound resulted from trauma. Repeated unsuccessful attempts were made to repair this wound with bandages, sutures and antibiotics.
i. What is the basic reason why the wound has not healed?
ii. How could this wound be repaired?

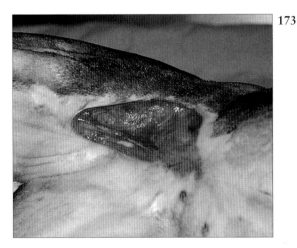

171 There are numerous ways to repair aural hematomas. (1) Simple drainage of the hematoma with a large gauge needle and bandage the ear. Multiple aspirations may be needed over a period of days to weeks (greater chance for recurrence). (2) Lance the hematoma on the concave surface of the pinna with a scalpel blade. Clot and fibrin are removed and mattress sutures are placed parallel to the incision. The incision edges are not reapposed and sutures should penetrate the full thickness of the ear. Knots are tied on the convex surface of the ear. The number of sutures is determined by the amount of dead space that must be closed. Postoperatively, ears may or may not be bandaged. The bandage is removed after 5–7 days and the sutures in 21 days. Other necessary protective devices that may be used are Elizabethan collars, neck shields or stockinette placed over the ears. (3) A sutureless technique involves elliptical incision over the swelling with removal of the clot and fibrin. The ear is bandaged over a roll of gauze or cast padding positioned on top of the head, making sure that the incision is open and exposed. The incision is covered with a dressing and changed as necessary. The incision heals by second intention and the ear is left bandaged for three weeks. (4) Placement of a bovine teat cannula through a stab incision into the hematoma. Fluid and fibrin are removed and the teat cannula is sutured in place with a figure-of-eight pattern. The owner is instructed to massage the ear twice daily and force fluid out of the hematoma. The cannula is left in place for three weeks and, as a minimum, an Elizabethan collar is placed to avoid self-trauma to the area.

172 i. Congenital urethrorectal fistula and large cystic calculus.
ii. Exposure to the fistula is by caudal ventral abdominal incision and pubic osteotomy. The catheterized fistula is easily identified by palpation, and it is excised after ligation of its attachments to the urethra and rectum with 4-0 synthetic absorbable material. Ventral cystotomy is performed to remove the cystic calculus (see **133**).
iii. Castration is recommended as the inheritance of this anomaly is uncertain.
iv. If left untreated, chronic cystitis will result in pyelonephritis. Other less serious sequelae include perianal dermatitis, urolith formation (as in this case) and chronic diarrhea.

173 i. Chronic skin defects occur in cats and the cause can be obscure. Pyogranulomatous panniculitis caused by mycobacterial infection, abscesses from bite wounds, indolent ulcers and other lesions are described. In this cat, biopsies and cultures did not identify a cause. Wounds in the inguinal and axillary region are subject to movement and tension, and this likely caused the open non-healing wound in this cat.
ii. For all reconstructive procedures the surgeon should select the simplest and quickest procedure. Undermining and mobilization of skin adjacent to the wound is rarely successful in this area. Free skin grafts are easier and more successful in cats than in dogs, and a graft could be used. An axial pattern flap from the opposite superficial epigastric artery or from the ipsilateral deep circumflex iliac artery should be successful. A simpler technique is an advancement or transposition flap. Skin fold advancement flaps in this region have been described recently. This author (D.E. Johnston) prefers a transposition flap of readily available skin craniodorsal to the wound.

174 With regard to the repair of the wound in the cat in 173, describe in detail the selected method.

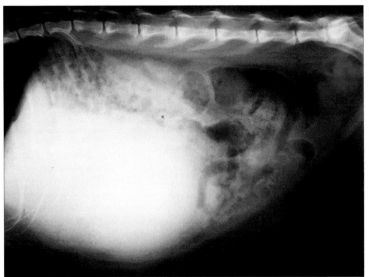

175a

175 A right lateral abdominal radiograph of a 12-year-old, domestic shorthair cat (175a) and the result of an exploratory laparotomy (175b) are shown.

i. Give your differential diagnoses for primary liver tumors in the cat.
ii. Describe two partial liver lobe resection techniques.
iii. How much of the liver can be resected without significant clinical dysfunction?

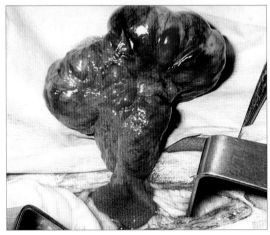

175b

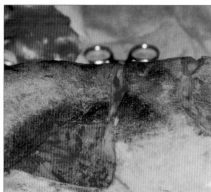

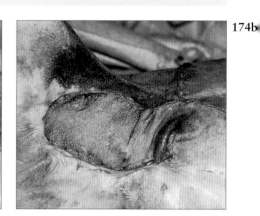

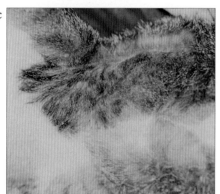

174 The cat is shown in lateral recumbency after the wound margins are debrided (174a). The transposition flap is outlined by incisions in the skin. Measurements were made to ensure the flap length and width correctly approximate the defect. The flap is transposed and sutured in place with subdermal absorbable simple interrupted sutures (174b). Since the subdermal fascia is strong and resistant to ischemic necrosis, simple interrupted skin sutures are inserted if needed; they were not needed in this case.

Flaps are not transposed beyond 90° to avoid interference with blood supply. This flap is transposed to the maximum degree and this created some skin folds in the base of the flap. These folds disappear rapidly without treatment.

In all flaps taken from the body wall the pattern of hair growth in the flap resembles that of the donor site, as can be seen in this flap at one year (174c).

175 i. Hepatocellular adenoma, hepatocellular adenocarcinoma, bile duct adenocarcinoma, focal hepatic malignant lymphoma.
ii. Liver lobectomy can be performed using the finger-fracture or suture-fracture technique. An incision is made in the liver capsule. The liver parenchyma is separated by digital pressure to isolate the blood vessels and large intralobar bile ducts. The blood vessels and bile ducts are ligated. Alternatively, the liver lobe can be resected using a thoracoabdominal stapler to crush through the parenchyma and apply a line of staples for hemostasis.
iii. Up to 75% of a normal liver can be resected without clinical dysfunction.

176a
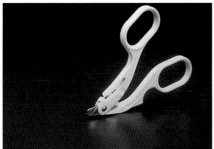

176b
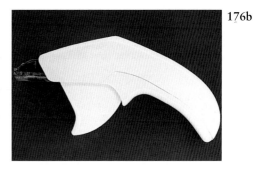

176 i. Identify this instrument (**176a**).
ii. Name two advantages to using this type of device (**176b**).
iii. Name two disadvantages to using this type of device.

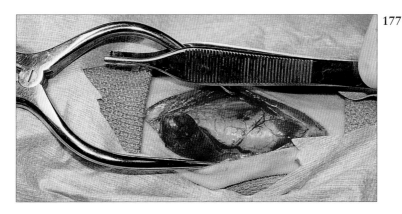
177

177 A 15-year-old, domestic shorthair cat was treated for hyperthyroidism by surgical removal of a thyroid adenoma (**177**). More than 90% of thyroid tumors in cats are adenomas and 70% occur bilaterally.
i. What are the benefits and complications of bilateral thyroidectomy?
ii. What are the different techniques used to perform bilateral thyroidectomy?
iii. What treatment options are available for feline hyperthyroidism other than surgery?

143

176, 177: Answers

176 i. Skin staple remover. The corresponding skin stapler is shown (176b). This type is disposable and can be sterilized in ethylene oxide.
ii. The major advantage of using skin staples for wound closure is the potential decrease in operating time. Stapling is the fastest method of closure for long skin incisions or lacerations. Decreased operating time, anesthetic administration and patient morbidity are resultant advantages of surgical stapling.
iii. Most surgical staples are made of 316 L stainless steel which causes minimal reaction; however, they produce artefacts in computed tomography and should not be used in animals that will undergo this procedure in the immediate postoperative period. Disadvantages of stapled skin closure include occasional malfunction (most manufacturers will replace any malfunctioning product) and increased cost. Staples are contraindicated if there is less than 4.0–6.5 mm between underlying bone or viscera and the skin to be closed.

177 i. Benefits of surgery include good success, low expense, requires less hospitalization and is more widely available than radioiodine therapy. Disadvantages are that hyperthyroid cats tend to be geriatric, cachectic and have concurrent cardiac or renal conditions making them poor candidates for anesthesia. Recurrent hyperthyroidism, hypocalcemia and hypothyroidism can develop and hyperactive ectopic thyroid tissue may be missed.
ii. Extracapsular. The cranial and caudal thyroid arteries are ligated and the gland removed with its capsule intact. The cranial parathyroid gland is spared, but there is usually damage to its blood supply. Recurrence of hyperthyroidism is low (less than 7%) but hypocalcemia occurs in up to 82% of patients.
Intracapsular. The capsule is opened and the thyroid gland is separated and removed from within. The cranial parathyroid gland and its blood supply are preserved. The capsule left behind may contain residual thyroid tissue, and an 8% recurrence rate of hyperthyroidism is reported. Hypocalcemia occurs in 15–22% of patients.
Modified extracapsular. The cranial thyroid artery is not ligated and the parathyroid gland is carefully spared. The thyroid gland and capsule is removed. Hyperthyroidism recurred in 4% of cases and hypocalcemia occurred in 23% of cases.
Modified intracapsular. After intracapsular thyroidectomy, the majority of the capsule is also removed except near the cranial parathyroid gland. This technique has a 34–47% incidence of hypocalcemia.
Staged bilateral thyroidectomy by any combination of the intracapsular, modified extracapsular and modified intracapsular methods. Thyroidectomies are separated by several weeks to minimize the incidence of hypocalcemia.
iii. Administration of methimazole, which blocks thyroid hormone synthesis but is not cytotoxic to neoplastic thyroid tissue. Administration is maintained for life or until alternative therapy is undertaken. Radioiodine therapy is a curative and safe method of treatment and is effective against ectopic thyroid tissue. However, it is often expensive, involves a 1–2 week period of hospitalization and is not widely available.

178 An 11-year-old, female Cocker Spaniel was presented for evaluation of an abundant, persistent serosanguinous vulvar discharge following estrus. The animal was not polydypsic/polyuric, and hemogram and serum biochemistry tests were normal, with the exception of a slight leukocytosis (WBC 12.5 × 10⁹/l (12,500/mm³)). Vaginal cytology showed large numbers of stratified squamous epithelial cells and serum progesterone concentration was 3.84 nmol/l (120 ng/dl). Abdominal ultrasound was performed and the area caudal to the left kidney is shown (178).
i. What round structure is being measured by the calibers in the image?
ii. What do the signs of proestrus reflect that is occurring physiologically?
iii. What is the diagnosis, and what treatment is advised?

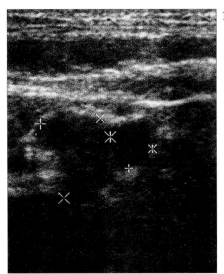

179 This is an oral view of a cystic mass of the right hemimandible in a 12-week-old Boxer (179). The patient was asymptomatic.
i. What is the tentative diagnosis?
ii. What test(s) would be most helpful in providing diagnostic information?
iii. What is the surgical treatment of choice for this lesion?

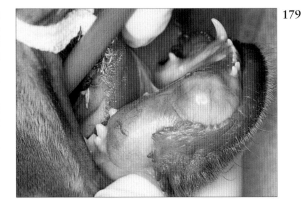

180 A 2-year-old Weimaraner is presented for reproductive evaluation after failure to breed. The owners report the dog would allow the male to mount, but would not allow intromission. The owners report no other abnormalities with the dog.
i. What two specific things should be done on physical examination to further evaluate this problem?
ii. You suspect a vaginal stricture. What two diagnostic tests are used to further define the abnormality?
iii. What is the treatment?

178 i. The left ovary with ovarian follicles that have not ruptured. Non-ovulation is confirmed by the animal's clinical signs and by the low serum progesterone concentration present. Cysts can be single or multiple and can affect one or both ovaries.
ii. The clinical signs of persistent proestrus are caused by estrogen production from the ovarian follicular cysts. These cysts occur from Graafian follicles that have not undergone atresia. Other commonly associated clinical signs include nymphomania, roaming, aggressiveness and mammary hyperplasia. Often these cysts are incidental findings at the time of routine ovariohysterectomy.
iii. Persistent ovarian follicles (or ovarian cysts) with production of estrogen. Treatment depends on the owners desire to maintain the reproductive function of the animal. If reproduction is of no concern to the owner, ovariohysterectomy is indicated; if breeding is desired, then medical management with GnRH or HCG is indicated to induce follicle rupture.

179 i. Tumor of dental epithelial origin.
ii. Radiographs of the mandible and analysis of fluid obtained from the mass using fine-needle aspiration. Radiographs showed bony lysis of the mandible and cytology did not indicate a neoplasm. In this patient, incisional biopsy was performed to determine the diagnosis (odontoma).
iii. Rostral unilateral hemimandibulectomy. Rarely, tumors of dental epithelial origin may resolve following curettage of the lesion. This latter procedure was performed in this patient at the time of incisional biopsy. The cystic mass recurred and rostral unilateral hemimandibulectomy was performed.

180 i. Digital examination of the vagina and rectal palpation. Vaginal palpation is performed first and is most useful to identify stenosis, persistent hymen, vaginal neoplasia or other intraluminal abnormalities. The most common location for congenital anomalies is the vestibulovaginal junction just cranial to the urethral papilla. Digital palpation is somewhat easier during estrus due to relaxation of the vagina. Rectal examination is most useful to define larger vaginal masses and extravaginal causes of obstruction.
ii. Vaginoscopy and contrast vaginography. Vaginoscopy is performed using a speculum, otoscope or endoscope. A small, single opening suggests annular stenosis; two small openings indicate a vertical septal band or double vagina are present. Vaginoscopy is helpful to evaluate the cranial part of the vagina, but lesions at the vestibulovaginal junction can be overlooked. Vaginography is performed by placing a Foley catheter and inflating the cuff just caudal to the vestibulovaginal junction. Radiopaque contrast is infused and radiographs are made. Vaginography may reveal vaginal septae, double vagina or vaginal masses, or it may outline a vaginal stricture.
iii. Surgical excision or vaginoplasty. The urethra is catheterized to identify its location and prevent accidental injury. Septal bands are best identified and excised by episiotomy; the mucosal defect is closed with absorbable suture. Annular constrictions are best exposed by a dorsal perineal approach to the vagina and managed by vaginoplasty (Y-U plasty or transverse closure of a longitudinal incision). It is important to evaluate the diameter of the vaginal lumen before wound closure. Breeding is not allowed for a minimum of two weeks.

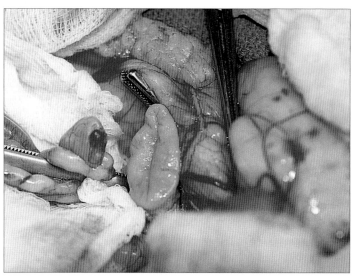

181a

181 This cat (181a) has been diagnosed with megacolon that is unresponsive to medical therapy. Subtotal colectomy is recommended for management.
i. What suture patterns are recommended for the colon?
ii. What suture material is appropriate for this anastomosis?
iii. What methods are available for managing the size disparity between ascending colon and rectum?

182 A six-year-old, female Basset-hound is presented with a soft doughy mass in the inguinal region (182). Vulvar enlargement typical of estrus is also noted.
i. What are the differential diagnoses for this mass?
ii. What are the anatomic, hormonal and metabolic factors that contribute to the occurrence of this problem?
iii. What two surgical approaches can be made for repair of this problem?

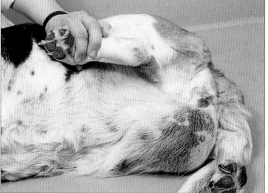

182

181, 182: Answers

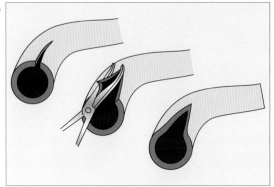

181 i. Because of the size disparity, difficulty suturing in the cranial pelvic canal and the need for distensibility and watertight apposition, simple interrupted sutures are commonly used. Sutures are placed to penetrate the submucosa and not the mucosal layer. In a canine model, simple interrupted appositional, crushing and inverting sutures had similar wound healing characteristics.

ii. Monofilament non-reactive suture on a taper needle is recommended. Polydioxanone, polypropylene and nylon incite minimal inflammation and are all good choices. Polydioxanone has the added advantage of being absorbable.

iii. Small variations in size are managed by placing sutures closer together on the small lumen side and slightly further apart on the large lumen side. Moderate variations in size are managed by cutting the smaller diameter bowel segment at an angle towards the antimesenteric side creating a larger lumen. Moderate to large disparities are managed by 'fish mouthing' the small diameter segment, incising the antimesenteric border (181b), or by suturing the segments routinely until the antimesenteric border of the small segment is reached and the remaining unsutured large segment is closed in an inverting pattern. Care is taken to ensure the anastomosis at the antimesenteric surface of the small segment is secure.

182 i. Differential diagnoses include inguinal hernia, abdominal wall hernia, seroma/hematoma and neoplasia. Diagnosis is determined by palpation (contents reducible), radiographs (tangential view of abdominal wall to look for discontinuity) and, if the above tests are inconclusive, fine-needle aspirate can be considered. The abnormality shown in this dog is an inguinal hernia.

ii. A large inguinal opening is considered the primary risk factor for herniation. Anatomically, females are predisposed because the inguinal canal is larger and shorter than in males; estrogen probably also plays a role by changing the strength and character of connective tissues, resulting in an enlarged canal. Most inguinal hernias occur in estral or pregnant bitches; an acquired inguinal hernia has not been reported in a spayed female. Weakness of the abdominal wall may also occur from an altered nutritional or metabolic state. Obese animals seem to be predisposed.

iii. Surgical repair can be by direct incision over the hernial sac and inguinal canal, or by ventral midline approach and reduction and closure of the inguinal canal from inside the abdomen. The midline approach avoids incising through mammary tissue in the lactating dog, and allows inspection of both inguinal canals. Midline incision is also a more familiar approach for most surgeons.

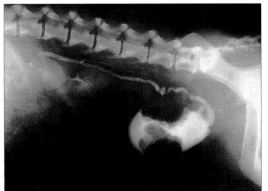

183a

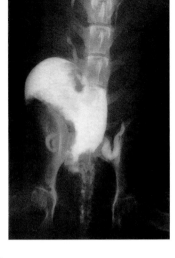

183b

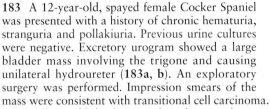

183 A 12-year-old, spayed female Cocker Spaniel was presented with a history of chronic hematuria, stranguria and pollakiuria. Previous urine cultures were negative. Excretory urogram showed a large bladder mass involving the trigone and causing unilateral hydroureter (183a, b). An exploratory surgery was performed. Impression smears of the mass were consistent with transitional cell carcinoma.

i. How else could the diagnosis have been made preoperatively?
ii. What are the surgical options if the tumor involves the trigone and both ureters? What options are available if the trigone is not involved?
iii. What are complications of urinary diversion techniques?

184 Name and describe the three components of the cardiac pacemaker pictured (184).

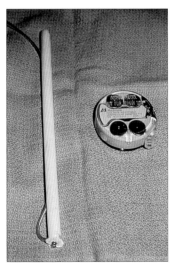

184

183 i. Preoperative diagnosis of a bladder mass can be made by ultrasound guided fine-needle aspiration. The clinician must beware of tumor seeding. Cells can also be collected by exfoliation into urine sediment either naturally or iatrogenically by large bore urethral catheter. However, this technique can be highly unreliable. Cystoscopy is most useful in determining the extent of tumor involvement and for collection of biopsy samples. It is the gold-standard for staging and diagnosis of bladder cancer in humans.
ii. Since most transitional cell carcinomas involve the trigone region, ureterocolonic anastomosis (UCA) is usually the surgical treatment of choice. If the trigone area is not involved, partial cystectomy or trigonal colonic anastomosis can be performed. Controversy continues over the role of surgery in the management of bladder cancer (see iii below).
iii. The most common complication of surgery is tumor recurrence. Urinary diversion procedures alone do not significantly increase the lifespan of patients. In a study of ten cases of UCA, nine dogs survived from 1–5 months after surgery. Other complications included pyelonephritis and hyperchloremic metabolic acidosis, hyperammonemia and elevated serum creatinine concentration. Electrolytes, acid-base status, renal biochemistry tests and urinalyses must be regularly monitored.

184 i. *Pulse generators* can be synchronous or asynchronous. Asynchronous pacemakers generate an impulse at a continuous, fixed rate and are not synchronized with the heart. They are relatively inexpensive, reliable, long lasting and are not very sensitive to external electromagnetic radiation. They may create competitive rhythms if the natural rhythm returns. Synchronous pacemakers sense spontaneous cardiac activity and either inhibit impulse generation, or deliver impulses synchronously during natural rhythms and asynchronously in the absence of natural rhythm, preventing occurrence of competitive rhythms. A three-letter code is used to identify the mode of generator operation. The first letter identifies the area of the heart being paced (A = atrium, V = ventricle, D = both). The second represents the area sensed (A = atrium, V = ventricle, O = neither). The third letter represents the mode of response (I = inhibited, T = triggered, O = neither). A VVI pacemaker is most commonly used in veterinary surgery.
Power sources can be mercury–zinc or lithium. Lithium cells have a longer life span (8–16 years compared with 3–6 for mercury–zinc) and fail by gradual decay; the mercury–zinc type fail by suddenly stopping.
Electrodes can be endocardial or epicardial. Endocardial (transvenous) electrodes are placed into the right ventricle through a branch of the cranial vena cava, and require a higher threshold potential to stimulate a beat. Epicardial–myocardial electrodes are either sutured or screwed into the myocardium of the ventricle. Less energy is required to initiate a heartbeat and the lifespan of the power source is increased. Either type of electrode may be unipolar or bipolar.

185 Describe a transdiaphragmatic approach for implantation of the cardiac pacemaker in 184.

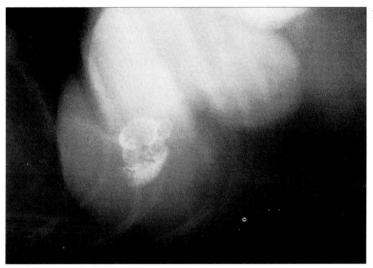

186a

186 A right lateral radiograph of the cranial abdomen of a ten-year-old, female Schnauzer is shown (186a).
i. What is the diagnosis?
ii. This disease is often insidious and asymptomatic in dogs. List the most common clinical signs in dogs that are symptomatic.
iii. The pathogenesis of this disease in dogs is unknown. Several causes have been proposed. Name the most likely ones.
iv. Describe the surgical therapeutic options, and give the therapy of choice.

185a 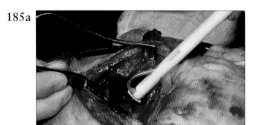 185b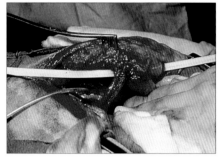

185c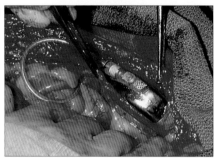

185 Transdiaphragmatic pacemaker implantation is performed via ventral midline celiotomy. The diaphragm is incised just left of midline and the pericardium identified and incised to expose the cardiac apex. A unipolar screw-type lead is implanted into the myocardium being careful to avoid the coronary arteries (**185a**). No sutures are required but the Dacron pledget must contact the epicardium to allow fibrous tissue ingrowth to anchor the electrode in place. The lead wire is connected to the pulse generator which when placed against the body wall becomes grounded, and the pacemaker begins to function. The lead may exit through the incision in the diaphragm or is passed between the diaphragm and body wall using the tunneler (**185b**). The diaphragm is closed and air is evacuated from the chest. The pulse generator is placed in a muscle pocket created between the muscles of the body wall (**185c**). This approach is rapid, cosmetic and less painful than a thoracotomy approach.

186b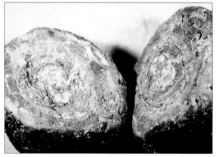

186 i. Cholelithiasis (**186b**).
ii. Vomiting, anorexia, weakness, polyuria/polydypsia, weight loss, icterus, fever and signs of abdominal pain are the most common clinical signs in dogs with symptomatic cholelithiasis.
iii. Proposed causes include trauma, biliary stasis, diet alterations, cholecystitis, and parasitic and bacterial biliary infection.
iv. The treatment for cholelithiasis is cholelithotomy via cholecystostomy, cholecystectomy or choledochotomy. Cholecystectomy is indicated in dogs with cholelithiasis and concurrent cholecystitis and should be regarded as therapy of choice.

187 An exploratory lapar-
otomy is performed on a five-
year-old cat with signs of
vomiting and anorexia for two
weeks (187).
i. What is this unusual abnormality?
ii. Biliary diversion techniques
can be used to circumvent bile
duct obstruction that cannot be
relieved. List the two methods
most commonly used.
iii. Describe technical considerations that improve the outcome of the surgical techniques
listed under (ii).

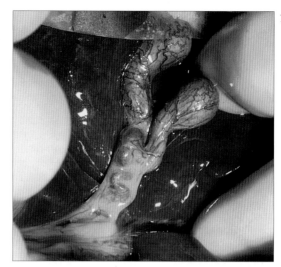

187

188 An 18-month-old Border
Collie crossbreed was presented for treatment of a nasal his-
tiocytoma. Cryosurgery was
used to treat this tumor (188).
i. To maximize cell destruction
what speeds should be used for
the freeze and thaw cycles, and
how many cycles are recommended?
ii. Describe the preparation of
a site for cryosurgery.
iii. List contraindications for
the use of cryosurgery.

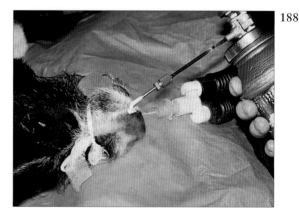

188

189 A six-week-old, male Boxer puppy with dyspnea is presented. On physical
examination you determine the puppy has dorsoventral compression of the chest
with a dorsal deviation of the sternum into the chest.
i. What is this condition called?
ii. Describe how the frontosagittal index and the vertebral index are determined.
iii. How are these indices used?
iv. Describe the technique that is currently recommended for treatment of this
condition.

187 i. Vesica duplex (double gall-bladder).
ii. Cholecystoduodenostomy and cholecystojejunostomy.
iii. The gall-bladder should be mobilized from its hepatic fossa to decrease tension at the stoma site. Stoma sizes of 2.5–4 cm have been recommended to prevent obstruction caused by contraction of the stoma during maturation of the wound. Spillage of bile and duodenal contents should be prevented during the surgery. Proper suture placement using a mucosal apposition technique and oversewing the serosa will prevent leakage and subsequent peritonitis.

188 i. Two cycles of rapid freezing (to -20°C/-4°F or cooler) and slow thawing are recommended to achieve optimal cell destruction. Rapid freezing results in small intracellular ice crystals which cause rupture of cell membranes. Large ice crystals, which cause cell damage by their size alone, form during a slow thaw.
ii. Preparation of the surgical patient is not as involved as for traditional surgery. Hair is clipped around the lesion to allow easier visualization of the ice ball and recognition of run-off of liquid nitrogen. Skin is cleaned if needles are to be used; however, sterility is not necessary. When a freeze is induced by spraying liquid nitrogen onto a lesion (as opposed to freezing by touching a probe to a lesion) surrounding tissues are protected by a thick layer of petroleum jelly.
iii. Contraindications for cryosurgery include mast cell tumors and tumors with bone involvement. Mast cells release heparin and histamine when lysed. Cancellous bone does not freeze well and cortical bone becomes weakened after freezing and can form a sequestrum. Large vessels that pass through treated tissue are ligated preoperatively to prevent hemorrhage when the eshcar sloughs.

189 i. Pectus excavatum.
ii. Frontosagittal index: chest width measured across the 10th thoracic vertebra on a ventrodorsal radiograph divided by the distance between the sternal deformity and ventral aspect of the closest vertebral body measured from the lateral radiograph. Vertebral index: distance from the dorsal surface of the vertebral bodies to the nearest point of the sternal defect as measured from a lateral radiograph divided by the diameter of the same vertebral body.
iii. A frontosagittal index of <2 and vertebral index of >9 is considered mild pectus excavatum. A frontosagittal index of 2.0–3.0 and a vertebral index of 6.0–9.0 are considered moderate and a frontosagittal index of >3.0 and a vertebral index of >9.0 are considered severe pectus excavatum. The severity of pectus excavatum is assessed using these indices. Surgery is indicated based on severity and the presence of clinical signs. These indices are also useful to determine improvement postoperatively.
iv. An external splint of a thermoplastic (VTP [IMEX Veterinary Inc.] or Orthoplast [Johnson and Johnson]) is cut and molded to a normal shape of the patient's chest. Holes are created in the splint separated by a distance slightly greater than the width of the sternebrae. Under general anesthesia, sutures are placed around the sternebra and through the holes in the splint. They are tightened to pull the sternum and chest to conform to the splint and are tied with bows so they may be adjusted as needed postoperatively. The bows are taped to the splint for security. The splint is left in place for 6–14 days. Contact irritation may occur under the splint.

190 Two small oronasal fistulae near the junction of the hard and soft palate are shown (190). The patient had multiple surgeries to close this area following the original trauma of foreign body (stick) penetration.
i. What are the expected clinical signs at this time?
ii. What is the likely reason for failure of previous surgeries?
iii. Describe a surgical repair that would avoid this problem.

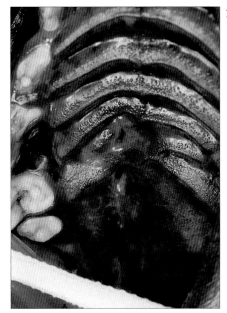

190

191 You are presented with a 12-week-old, male Weimaraner puppy with a history of regurgitation noticed shortly after the puppy was purchased from the breeder. On physical examination the puppy is thin but alert and active. The owners report that he does not regurgitate liquids. Survey radiographs of the chest and abdomen are normal. The barium swallow results are shown (191).
i. What is the most likely diagnosis?

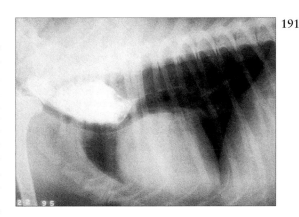
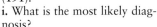

191

ii. Describe the pathophysiology of this condition.
iii. How should this dog be managed prior to surgery, and when should surgery be performed?
iv. Describe the surgical management of this condition.
v. What is the long-term prognosis for this dog, and how should it be managed post-operatively?

190, 191: Answers

190 **i.** Clinical signs in this dog were mild, intermittent sneezing and gagging especially after drinking water. Since this lesion is caudal, the dog did not have clinical signs of rhinitis.

ii. Inappropriate tension at the surgery site. Failure to immobilize tissues adequately and decrease tension at the suture line is the primary reason for failure of cleft palate and oronasal fistula repair. The prognosis is good if excessive tension is prevented.

iii. The bridge of tissue between the two defects was excised. The perimeter of the defect was incised to provide two separate layers. Relief incisions of the oral mucosa were made from the middle of the soft palate, along the dental arcade, and ending between the second and third premolars. Submucosal dissection plane was developed with a perisoteal elevator resulting in bilateral contiguous soft palate mucosa and hard palate mucoperiosteal flaps. Dissection and undermining was performed from the lateral aspects (relief incisions) to the midline defect. Thus, in effect, two bipedicle mucosal flaps were developed with the midline component consisting of the defect. The defect was then sutured in two layers (nasopharyngeal mucosa, oral mucosa) using simple interrupted polyglactin 910. The knots of the oral suture line were buried to prevent licking causing knot disruption.

191 **i.** Vascular ring anomaly. Persistent right aortic arch is most likely. A breed pre-disposition is identified for Weimaraners, Great Danes, Irish Setters and Doberman Pinschers.

ii. Persistent right aortic arch results from failure of the left aortic arch to develop as the dominant structure in the fetus; instead, the right aortic arch develops. Cardio-vascular physiology is normal but the ligamentum arteriosum (ductus arteriosus of the fetus) connects the right-sided aorta to the pulmonary artery creating the vascular ring entrapping the esophagus and trachea. The primary clinical sign is regurgitation at weaning. Emaciation and aspiration pneumonia may occur secondarily.

iii. Surgery is performed as soon as possible. If aspiration pneumonia is present, it is treated first. If surgery is delayed, the esophagus may develop permanent loss of muscle tone and neurologic dysfunction. Prior to surgery, the puppy is fed a liquid or gruel diet (small amounts frequently, from an elevated position) which will pass through the vascular ring.

iv. Surgery involves transection of the ligamentum arteriosum and freeing the esophagus from its entrapment within the vascular ring. The ligamentum arteriosum, approached via left lateral 4th intercostal thoracotomy, is identified caudal to the esophageal dilation and dissected free from attachments to the esophagus. Because it can be patent, the ligament is double ligated and transected between ligatures. A large orogastric tube is inserted into the esophagus and passed through the constricted area; any tissue preventing distension is dissected free allowing the tube to pass easily.

v. Prognosis with early surgical treatment is good. The longer surgery is delayed, the poorer the prognosis. Postoperative management is identical to preoperative manage-ment. Four weeks following surgery the puppy is gradually returned to a normal diet. If regurgitation occurs, a barium swallow is repeated to determine the status of the esophagus.

192 Name two different modalities for vascular ligation.

193 This is a ventrodorsal view of a cranial abdominal radiograph (**193**).
i. What diagnostic study has been performed, and what is the diagnosis?
ii. What other diagnostic tests could have been performed to obtain a definitive diagnosis?
iii. Name the potential postoperative complications associated with the surgical correction of this disease.

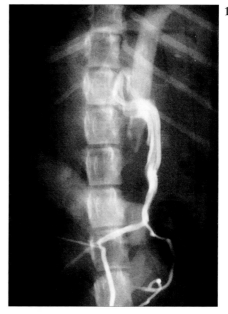
193

194 This is an oral view of the sublingual area in a five-year-old, mixed-breed dog (**194**). The patient has a history of anorexia and intermittent vomiting. The patient was undergoing an exploratory laparotomy when the sublingual area was examined.
i. What diagnostic test(s) indicated surgery was necessary?
ii. Why was the sublingual area specifically examined?
iii. If the patient had not had clinical signs of gastrointestinal disease, name an additional differential diagnoses?

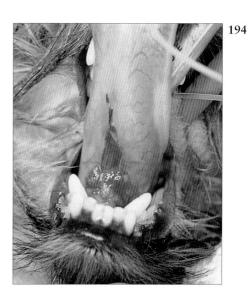
194

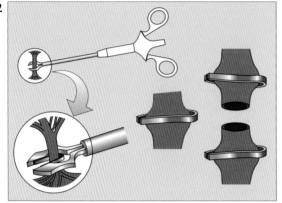

192 Vascular ligation can be performed with sutures or surgical staples. Suture patterns acceptable for ligation include a simple ligature, Halstead transfixation ligature, modified transfixation ligature and tissue ligature. Double ligatures are recommended for large isolated vessels, especially arteries. Knot security is inversely proportional to suture diameter; therefore the smallest suture providing adequate strength is used.

Vascular clips are an alternative for ligation of small vessels (**192**). Advantages are they can be applied rapidly and accurately, easily applied in poorly accessible areas where suture ligation is difficult, and metal clips are radiopaque and can serve as landmarks of the surgical site on radiographs. The disadvantage is that clips are more easily dislodged, especially if there is tissue manipulation after placement. To apply clips, dissect as much surrounding tissue as possible from the vessel to be occluded. The diameter of the vessel to be ligated should be no larger that two-thirds the length of the clip. The vascular clip is applied several millimeters from the cut end of the vessel to avoid slippage. An artery and its accompanying vein are clipped separately.

193 i. Jejunal vein portography. Extrahepatic portosystemic shunt from the portal vein to the caudal vena cava. The extrahepatic location of the shunt is deduced from the fact that the shunt is located caudal to the T13 vertebral body.
ii. Splenoportography; cranial mesenteric portography; celiac arteriography; intravenous, transcolonic, and intrasplenic nuclear scintigraphy. All imaging studies are diagnostic of portosystemic shunt if contrast material (radiopaque or nuclear) is detected to bypass the liver and directly enter the systemic circulation.
iii. Postoperative complications following shunt ligation include portal hypertension, portal vein thrombosis, ascites, delayed wound healing, hemorrhage, hypoglycemia, infection, seizures and death.

194 i. Abdominal radiographs and ultrasound showed 'pleating' of small bowel suggestive of a string foreign body.
ii. The sublingual area is always examined in patients with a string foreign body. This patient indeed had an intestinal string foreign body which could not be removed by enterotomy until the portion around the tongue had been cut. Intestinal string foreign body which is caught at the tongue will 'saw' into the frenulum causing inflammation and exuberant granulation tissue as in this dog.
iii. Squamous cell carcinoma can appear very similar.

195 An eight-year-old, male Great Pyrenees presents with a history of a gradual onset of weakness, lethargy and coughing. Recently, the owners noticed abdominal distension. On physical examination you determine there is ascites, and muffled heart sounds on thoracic auscultation. Radiographs reveal a dramatically enlarged cardiac silhouette. A cardiac ultrasound is shown (195).

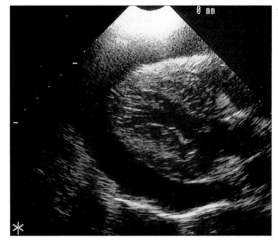

i. What is your sonographic diagnosis?

You collect a sample for cytology and it consists of a sterile, non-clotting fluid with erythrocytes, macrophages and reactive mesothelial cells. There is no evidence of neoplasia on ultrasound examination or on cytologic evaluation.

ii. What is your definitive diagnosis?
iii. What treatment is recommended for this condition?
iv. What histologic changes would you expect to find?
v. What is the long-term prognosis with surgical management?

196 This is a lateral radiograph of a three-year-old, female domestic shorthair cat made at the local emergency clinic (196a). The cat is your patient and was hit by a car the night before, treated at the emergency clinic and referred to you for further treatment. The cat is painful and somewhat dyspneic.

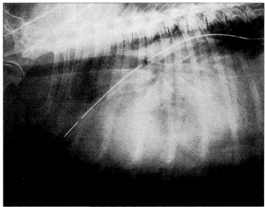

i. What is your diagnosis based on this radiograph?
ii. What treatment would you recommend?

195 i. Pericardial effusion. The source and character of effusion cannot be determined without further testing.
ii. In the absence of infectious or neoplastic disease, a definitive diagnosis of idiopathic hemorrhagic pericardial effusion (IHPE) is made based on cytology.
iii. Treatment for IHPE is intermittent pericardiocentesis, or total or partial pericardiectomy. Many clinicians attempt pericardiocentesis and recommend pericardiectomy if the condition recurs. The disadvantage of pericardiocentesis is that acute cardiac tamponade with fatal consequences may occur at any time. Pericardiectomy (total or subtotal) removes much or all of the diseased pericardium and allows any produced to drain into the thoracic cavity and be absorbed without risk of tamponade. This procedure is contraindicated in cases of infectious pericarditis.
iv. Fibrous connective tissue and fibrin tag deposition on the parietal pericardium. The cardiac surface of the parietal pericardium usually has the most active lesions. Changes can include hemorrhage, congestion, neovascularization, inflammation and fibroplasia. Lymphocytes and plasma cells predominate though macrophages are prominent in some cases. Marked mesothelial proliferation may also be present.
v. Though the etiology remains unknown, the prognosis is good; most dogs are normal following pericardiectomy.

196b

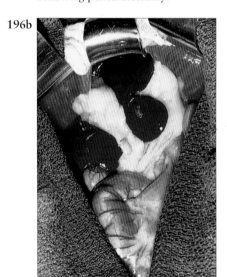

196 i. Traumatic diaphragmatic hernia. The heart and lungs are displaced dorsally by what appears to be the liver. There is no distinct separation between the abdomen and thorax. A thoracotomy tube has been placed.
ii. First, the patient is stabilized and treated for shock. High mortality rates occur when surgery is performed within the first 24 hours (33%) due to shock, organ failure and the stress of anesthesia and surgery. Surgery (diaphragmatic herniorrhaphy) is performed as soon as the patient is stable.

Anesthesia is induced quickly, the patient intubated, and ventilation controlled until the hernia is repaired and negative pressure established in the pleural space. For acute hernia, a ventral midline celiotomy is recommended (196b). Other approaches (a ninth intercostal thoracotomy, a median sternotomy and a transsternal thoracotomy) are indicated only if adhesions are present. Abdominal viscera are returned to their normal position. A malleable retractor is used to keep viscera reduced allowing inspection and closure of the diaphragm. Even with chronic tears, it is not necessary to debride the edges of the hernia. An absorbable material such as polygalactin 910 or polydioxanone is preferred and the pattern may be either continuous or interrupted. Closure is initiated dorsal (deep) and continued ventral. A chest tube is placed for 24–48 hours postoperatively.

197 With regard to the cat in 196 with traumatic diaphragmatic hernia:
i. Which side, if either, is more commonly involved?
ii. What are the major postoperative complications associated with this procedure? Discuss re-expansion pulmonary edema.

198 An eight-year-old, spayed female Cocker Spaniel is presented for treatment of chronic otitis externa. The dog has had otitis for years and in the past, medical management would palliate the dog. Currently the dog is so painful she will not allow the owners to treat the ears, and recent response to medical therapy has been poor.
i. What are the surgical treatments for chronic otitis externa?
ii. What criteria are used to choose the appropriate procedure?
iii. What additional diagnostic tests can be performed before surgery to fully evaluate the ears?

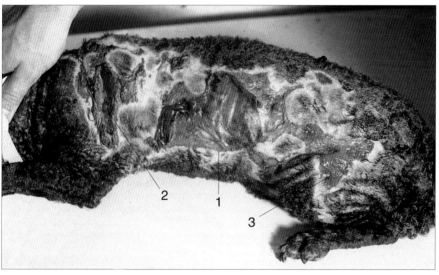

199

199 This five-year-old, mixed-breed dog (199) received a burn from a heating pad during surgery approximately three months ago. The dog is systemically healthy and there is no evidence of infection, electrolyte abnormalities, protein loss, etc. In addition to the areas of hair loss and epithelialization, there are three wounds; the largest of these is in the caudal thoracic and cranial abdominal area and is a square wound almost entirely covered with a tightly adherent dried eschar (1). Cranial to this wound over the shoulder and upper arm is a second major wound also covered with an adherent dried eschar (2). The third is the open granulating wound over the stifle and thigh (3). Is this a typical burn wound? Describe the nature of these individual wounds.

197 i. Reports vary, but when put together there is an even distribution between right-sided and left-sided diaphragmatic hernias. In dogs, about 40% have peripheral tears, 40% have central tears and 20% have a combination. In cats, about 60% have peripheral tears, 20% have central tears and 20% have a combination.
ii. Hemothorax, pneumothorax, hypoventilation due to pain, ascites from increased hepatic venous pressure and re-expansion pulmonary edema. Re-expansion edema occurs when lung, atelectatic for a prolonged period, is rapidly re-expanded. Chronically atalectatic lung should be gradually reinflated. If the lung does not inflate with pressures of 20–30 cmH$_2$O, further attempts are not made. A chest tube is placed and the lung expanded gradually over hours or days. Corticosteroids may have a protective role in preventing pulmonary edema. Treatment is with ventilation and diuretics but is frequently unrewarding.

198 i. *Lateral ear canal resection* exposes the vertical and horizontal canals via excision of the lateral portion of the vertical cartilage. It is used to relieve stenosis of the vertical canal, and expose the horizontal canal improving drainage, air circulation, and application of topical medications.
  Vertical canal resection is performed if severe chronic otitis is limited to the vertical canal or a small tumor or polyp is present. The horizontal canal mucosa is apposed to the skin.
  Total ear ablation is performed to remove the entire cartilaginous ear canal. It is most often combined with lateral bulla osteotomy since otitis media is a common complication of severe, chronic otitis externa.
ii. Criteria used to choose the appropriate procedure are the extent and severity of disease. Mild to moderate chronic otitis externa without marked epithelial hyperplasia often responds better to medical therapy after lateral ear canal resection. Lateral canal resection is indicated only if the horizontal canal is patent. If the vertical canal is severely affected or a tumor is present, and the horizontal canal is patent, vertical ear canal ablation is indicated. Complete ear canal ablation is indicated if hyperplastic or neoplastic tissue extends to the horizontal canal or bulla.
iii. To properly determine the severity and extent of ear disease, physical, neurologic and otoscopic (may need to be performed after anesthesia) examinations are performed. Radiographs are made of the bullae, including left and right lateral oblique views, and an open-mouth rostrocaudal view. Changes seen include calcification of the external ear canal, thickening of the bullae walls and increased opacity of the bullae chambers.

199 Burns from heating devices used during surgery occur from prolonged contact with a moderate heat source. Burns usually occur with solid pad heating elements and very rarely with flowing warm water pads. Pad temperature should not exceed 42°C and immobile animals are moved regularly to avoid prolonged contact between one area of skin and the heat source. The limb wound (3) is a mixture of first, second and third degree burns. The first and second degree burns have healed, causing areas of hairlessness and epithelialization. All three third degree burns were originally covered with a coagulum of scab and dried skin. This eschar was removed from the hindlimb wound (3) and it is now healing by contraction and epithelialization. Because of adequate loose skin in this area, healing will be complete and contracture deformity will not occur. The other two wounds are covered with a leathery eschar which prevents wound contraction. Early in care, dried eschars are removed slowly by lifting the edges as much as the patient allows on a regular basis.

200 With regard to the dog in 199, what is the definitive therapy?

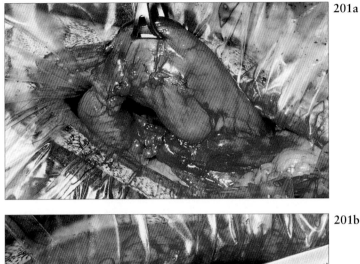

201a

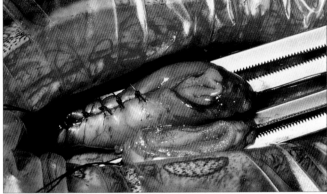

201b

201 A gastric outflow resection procedure is shown (201a, b).
i. Name the procedure.
ii. Describe an alternative technique.
iii. What are the complications associated with both techniques?

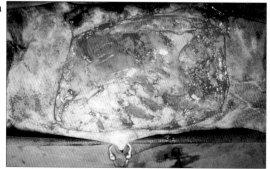

200a

200 The eschar in the cranial wound is excised and this wound is sutured easily. The caudal granulating wound is healing and is allowed to continue to do so. Available skin is saved for the major wound in the middle. The eschar in the middle wound is excised, creating a square defect on the lateral body wall (200a). Loose skin on the right side is easily transferred to the left by means of a bipedicle advancement flap or H-plasty. Four incisions are required: two incisions continue the sides of the square defect dorsally over the back of the dog and two incisions are made in the same manner ventrally under the abdomen. The flaps are undermined, leaving loose subcutaneous tissue and large vessels attached to the skin to preserve blood supply. The incisions are extended and undermining is

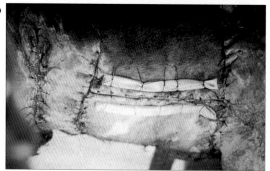

200b

continued until the free edges of the flaps can be advanced across the defect (200b). Divergence of the incisions as they are made prevents the base of the flap becoming narrowed when it is advanced. Survival of a bipedicle flap is dependent on random blood vessels entering the flap, and in this case is almost assured because of the many vessels over the trunk and the width to length ratio of the flaps is more than 1:1. If the width to length ratio is less, an attempt is made to devise an axial pattern flap instead.

201 i. Pylorectomy and gastroduodenostomy (Billroth I).
ii. Gastrojejunostomy (Billroth II). Following pylorectomy the pyloric and antral stumps are closed using an inverted two-layer suture pattern. Full-thickness longitudinal incisions are made in the stomach and jejunum. The jejunum and stomach are then sutured together using a two-layer closure technique.
iii. Incisional leakage and dehiscence, hemorrhage, pancreatic or common bile duct injury, persistent gastric outflow obstruction, marginal ulceration and stricture of the stoma.

202 The buried continuous intradermal closure technique (also called subcuticular or intradermal pattern) has gained popularity in veterinary surgical procedures. In which of the following cases is this suture pattern appropriate as an alternative to skin sutures?
(a) A five-year-old, male Labrador Retriever undergoing a routine castration.
(b) A ten-month-old, male Doberman Pinscher with an infected skin laceration requiring debridement and closure.
(c) A six-month-old, female Siamese undergoing a routine ovariohysterectomy.
(d) A ten-year-old Husky with a large mass at the lateral aspect of the stifle.

203a 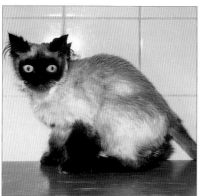 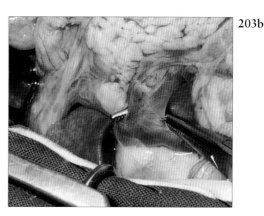 203b

203 A seven-month-old cat is presented with intermittent behavioral and neurological abnormalities (203a). The abdominal cavity of this cat during exploratory laparotomy is shown (203b).
i. What is the diagnosis?
ii. Describe the surgical therapy.
iii. What is the prognosis following surgery?

204 A 12-year-old, female Husky crossbreed was presented for treatment of a tonsillar mass. A carbon dioxide (CO_2) laser was used to excise the tumor.
i. What are advantages and disadvantages of CO_2 laser excision compared with scalpel excision?
ii. What are the patient safety precautions illustrated (204)? Name another safety precaution not shown.
iii. What safety precautions are taken by the surgeon and assistants?

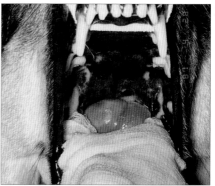 204

202 Both (a) and (c) are appropriate cases for using intradermal closure pattern alone. This closure pattern is best not used alone if wound edges are under tension, in contaminated or infected wounds, or wounds requiring drainage. The buried continuous intradermal closure technique is ideal for elective veterinary surgical procedures because it eliminates the need for suture removal. Absorbable, inert, light-colored sutures with a swaged needle are preferred. Appropriate sizes range from 3-0 to 6-0, depending on the incision location and cosmetic consideration; 4-0 size is usually preferred. Sutures should be placed superficial enough to hold skin edges together but deep enough so that they are covered by a healthy epithelial layer. Knots are buried entirely beneath the dermis to avoid interference with dermal coaptation and suture extrusion.

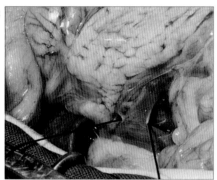

203c

203 i. Extrahepatic portosystemic shunt (see **193**).
ii. The anomalous vessel is identified and a ligature is placed as close to the vena cava as possible (**203c**). Portal vein pressure is monitored during attenuation of the vessel, and visual inspection of the splanchnic viscera is used to evaluate circulation and look for signs of passive congestion. The anomalous vessel is partially or totally closed, depending on the rise in portal pressure and the quality of visceral perfusion. More recently, reports of shunt occlusion using an ameroid ring have shown good results with limited morbidity and mortality (see **135**).
iii. The prognosis following surgery for portosystemic shunts in cats is less favorable than in dogs because postoperative improvement is less predictable. Persistence or relapse of clinical signs after initial improvement is common and is caused in some cases by development of multiple acquired portosystemic shunts after surgery.

204 i. The CO_2 laser controls hemorrhage better than scalpel surgery. This is desirable in vascular areas such as the oral cavity, where physical access is limited, and in patients with coagulopathies. The CO_2 laser seals lymphatics, theoretically minimizing dissemination of tumor cells during surgery. Disadvantages of CO_2 laser include cost of equipment and specialized training of staff.
ii. The endotracheal tube is covered with crinkled aluminum foil to prevent laser penetration and potential ignition of gas vapors and plastic. Surrounding soft tissues are protected from reflections with saline soaked gauzes. Not shown is suction for removal of the plume (smoke) that can cause respiratory irritation of both patient and surgeon. It is possible for viral particles and viable DNA from the target tissue to be transported in the plume.
iii. Safety glasses are necessary to protect all personnel from stray laser reflections that can cause ocular damage. A CO_2 fire extinguisher and a bucket of water for quenching flaming drapes, etc. should be available. A laser emblem logo is posted outside the operating room to alert staff of potential danger and to advise personnel entering the room that eye protection must be worn. Personnel must be trained in the safe operation of laser equipment before it is used.

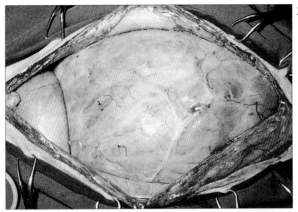

205a

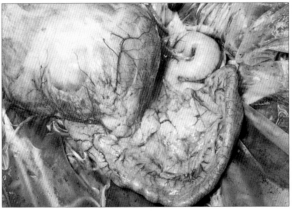

205b

205 A seven-year-old, male Golden Retriever is presented with a history of acute vomiting, depression, anorexia and diarrhea. A large, painful mass was detected by abdominal palpation. The findings during abdominal exploration are shown (205a, b).
i. What are the differential diagnoses?
ii. What is the recommended therapy for this dog?
iii. Partial pancreatectomy can be performed by two techniques. Name these techniques and their advantages.

206 When considering renal biopsy to gain a specific diagnosis:
i. What are some important contraindications, complications and perioperative considerations?
ii. Which biopsy needle is most commonly used and why?
iii. Name four different approaches to the kidneys, and the advantages and disadvantages of each.

167

205, 206: Answers

205 i. Pancreatic abscess, pancreatic pseudocyst, pancreatic neoplasm.
ii. Removal of the mass by partial pancreatectomy. Debridement and open abdominal drainage is recommended in septic dogs with pancreatic abscesses. Jejunostomy feeding tube should be placed if prolonged anorexia or vomiting is anticipated after surgery.
iii. The dissection and ligation technique and the suture-fracture technique. The former procedure allows precise identification and ligation of vessels and ducts, and causes less inflammatory reaction. The latter procedure is less precise but requires less time. It is more useful for resection of a distal limb of the pancreas.

206 i. Contraindications for renal biopsy include coagulopathies, marked hydronephrosis, suspected abscess, shrunken end-stage kidneys, and clinicians unfamiliar with the technique or lacking appropriate equipment. Complications include non-diagnostic specimens, gross or microscopic hematuria (3%), hemorrhagic shock (3%) and hydronephrosis from renal pelvis obstruction by blood clots. Platelet count, coagulation time and preferably renal sonography are evaluated before biopsy.

ii. The disposable (reusable as long as sharpness is satisfactory) Vim Tru-Cut style biopsy needle (206). The closed needle is advanced to the kidney capsule, and directed away from the pelvis. At least two samples are obtained. Tangential cutting needle cores or a thin wedge biopsy taken from the kidney pole provides good samples of cortex and medulla with minimal risk to renal pelvis. If the approach allows, pressure is applied to the biopsy site for 2–5 minutes. Eight to twelve hours of diuresis after biopsy helps prevent formation of blood clots in the renal pelvis. Automated biopsy needles such as the one shown are now available; these render manual immobilization of the kidney unnecessary.

iii. A blind percutaneous approach is outdated due to inadequate lesion localization, renal immobilization, hemostasis and specimen acquisition success rate. Key hole technique is simple and reliable, but allows access to only one kidney at a time. This approach is made by a 45° skin incision at the craniodorsal corner where the last rib meets the sublumbar musculature. Muscles are separated along the axis of their fibers and the peritoneum incised. A finger is inserted to palpate and stabilize the kidney for percutaneous cutting needle biopsy.

Ventral midline laparotomy provides access to both kidneys and is preferred when exploration of the entire urinary tract (or abdomen) is needed.

Percutaneous ultrasound-guided biopsy using an automated cutting needle device can be performed under sedation. Precise location of the area to biopsy is provided and morbidity is minimal. Ultrasound examination also allows evaluation of the entire urinary tract.

207a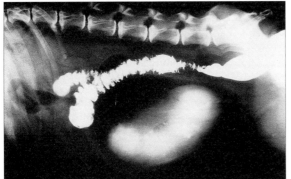

207b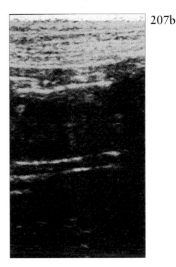

207 A seven-year-old, female German Shepherd Dog presented for consultation was previously diagnosed with acute cystitis. Its last estrus was nine weeks ago. On clinical examination a seropurulent vulvar secretion was observed. A contrast radiographic study is shown (207a) together with an ultrasound image of the patient's caudal abdomen (207b).
i. What contrast techniques have been used?
ii. Is the appearance of the studied organs normal?
iii. What is the diagnosis?

208 A nine-year-old, male Labrador Retriever is presented on emergency for acute onset of dyspnea. The owners report the dog was breathing heavily all day, but this evening became much worse. On presentation the dog has marked inspiratory stridor and is cyanotic. Body temperature is 40.6°C (105°F).
i. Where is the location of the obstruction, and what is the most likely cause?
ii. What emergency treatment is required?
iii. Briefly describe the needed emergency surgical procedure.

209 i. What are these instruments (209a)?
ii. Name three procedures that are performed using these instruments.

209a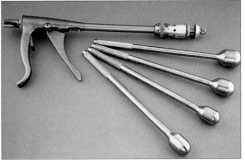

207 i. Double contrast hysterography (air and iodine contrast) and double contrast cystography. The contrast material used was Iohexol (300 mg I/ml) at a dose of 1 ml/kg body weight.
ii. No. The bladder wall is thickened and its outline irregular. The uterine outline is irregular in both horns. Urinalysis showed inflammatory sediment, and urine culture grew *Escherichia coli*. Corpora lutea were seen on ultrasound examination of the ovaries and serum progesterone concentration was 80 nmol/l (25 ng/ml).
iii. Cystitis and cystic endometrial hyperplasia. Treatment for cystitis is antibiotic therapy based on urine culture and sensitivity. Treatment for cystic endometrial hyperplasia, if symptomatic, is ovariohysterectomy or perhaps chemical luteolysis by prostaglandin therapy.

208 i. Inspiratory stridor is caused by upper airway obstruction. Given signalment, history and physical examination findings, laryngeal paralysis is likely.
ii. Emergency therapy consists of cooling the animal (alcohol/water bath, fan, fluids), decreasing laryngeal inflammation and edema with corticosteroids, and breaking the 'stress–dyspnea' cycle with sedation and oxygen therapy. If the animal decompensates in spite of medical treatment or presents in a life-threatening condition, as this dog is, a patent airway is established by temporary tracheostomy.
iii. Depending on the degree of urgency, the patient is best prepared and draped for aseptic surgery. In critical cases the hair is clipped and skin only swabbed with antiseptic. A ventral midline approach is made to the larynx. The annular ligament is transected one-half to two-thirds the circumference of the trachea between two rings (usually rings 3 and 4) being careful not to damage the recurrent laryngeal nerves. Alternatively, a vertical incision can be made through the tracheal rings. The tube is placed and secured with umbilical tape around the neck. A long, non-absorbable stay suture is placed around the distal tracheostomy ring and left in place to expose the trachea by applying traction, in the event the tube needs to be replaced urgently. Muscle, subcutis and skin are closed to the level of the tube. Antiseptic ointment is placed at the open incision site.

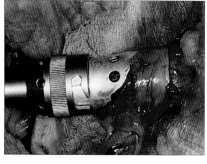

209b

209 i. End-to-end anastomosis (EEA) stapling instrument (United States Surgical Corporation, Norwalk, CT) and corresponding ovoid sizers. The EEA applies a circular double row of staples, creating a true two-layer inverting anastomosis. A circular blade within the cartridge simultaneously cuts the redundant 'doughnut-shaped' ring of tissue from each bowel end to create a new lumen. The ovoid sizers are used to determine lumenal diameter and hence which size EEA cartridge is used.
ii. Common uses of the EEA stapler include: colorectal resection and anastomosis (**209b**), end-to-end gastroduodenostomy, end-to-side gastroesophageal anastomosis, and esophageal and colonic anastomoses.

210 A lethargic nine-year-old, male German Shepherd Dog is presented with abdominal distension and an abdominal mass. Plain radiography confirms spleno-megaly and a splenectomy is performed. The enlarged spleen is shown (**210**).
i. Name the different causes of localized splenomegaly.
ii. What laboratory tests should be per-formed before surgery?
iii. List four predictors of splenic neo-plasia.
iv. A malignant tumor derived from blood vessels is diagnosed by histologic examination. What is the prognosis?

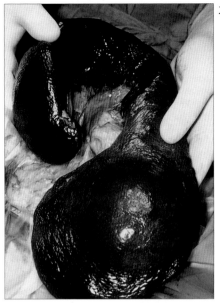

210

211 A 12-year-old, female Lhasa Apso is admitted to your hospital for evaluation of chronic weight loss, vomiting and diarrhea. On presentation, the dog is depressed, 12% dehydrated, tachycardic, has weak femoral pulses and its respirations are labored. Body temperature is 40.6°C (105°F) and the abdomen is tense and painful. Hemogram and serum chemistry abnormalities include: WBC 42 × 10⁹/l (42,000/mm³); PCV 0.52 l/l (52%); albumin 19.0 g/l (1.9 g/dl); platelets 75 × 10⁹/l (75,000/mm³); urea 7.97 mmol/l (BUN 48.0 mg/dl); glucose 2.9 mmol/l (52 mg/dl). Elevations of serum creatinine, alkaline phosphatase, bilirubin, amylase and lipase are noted, as well as hypokalemia and hypochloremia. Abdominocentesis recovers purulent fluid (WBC 55 × 10⁹/l (55,000/mm³)), with degenerative neutrophils and bacteria present. Amylase and lipase concentrations in the fluid are greater than those found in the serum. On sonography a pancreatic mass with a mixed echo pattern, possibly an abscess, is seen. Suspecting septic shock from a pancreatic abscess, you initiate treatment.
i. What are the fluid therapy options for acute restoration of intravascular volume? Which is preferred for patients in septic shock, and why?
ii. Thoracic radiographs show mild pulmonary edema and moderate plural effusion. This patient has no history of cardiopulmonary disease. What changes in the labora-tory values could account for these findings, and why? What treatment is used to reverse this process?
iii. Arterial blood gas analysis indicates metabolic acidosis is present. Why does this occur in septic shock, and how is it treated?
iv. Exploratory laparotomy is performed and a pancreatic abscess is diagnosed. Post-operatively, what steps besides i/v crystalloid therapy are considered to support this patient nutritionally?

210 i. Splenomegaly can be caused by primary neoplasia (hemangiosarcoma, lympho-sarcoma, leiomyosarcoma, fibrosarcoma, plasma cell tumor, mast cell tumor and hemangioma), metastic disease and non-neoplastic disease (hyperplasia and hematoma).
ii. Routine laboratory tests should include hemogram, BUN, creatinine and liver enzymes. Hemostasis should be investigated before surgery because splenic hemangio-sarcoma is associated with diffuse intravascular coagulation at the time of presenta-tion in up to 50% of cases.
iii. Anemia, nucleated red blood cells, abnormal red blood cell morphology and splenic rupture were found to be associated with a significantly greater chance of splenic neoplasia in dogs.
iv. A splenectomy is often life-saving in dogs with hemangiosarcoma, but a cure is seldom obtained. Hemangiosarcoma is associated with an average survival time of 2–3 months after splenectomy.

211 i. Fluid therapy options for this patient include: balanced electrolyte solutions such as lactated Ringer's or similar (90 ml/kg/hour); 7.5% saline (4–8 ml/kg); colloid therapy with dextran (dose 20 ml/kg) or hydroxyethyl starch (dose 20 ml/kg). Because large volumes of crystalloid solutions are required in septic shock to restore microcir-culation, concurrent use of colloids or hypertonic saline during resuscitation is recom-mended to reduce the amount of crystalloid required by 40–60%.
ii. Serum proteins, especially albumin, provide oncotic pressure in the normal animal. Hypoalbuminemia exacerbates fluid leakage into the interstitium, promoting peripheral and pulmonary edema. Administration of colloids can reduce or prevent edema from forming. When albumin concentration is less than 20 g/l, fresh frozen plasma or albumin are the colloids of choice. Once serum albumin is above 20 g/l, synthetic colloids such as dextran 70 or hydroxyethyl starch are used. The oncotic activity of dextran is stronger but not as long lasting as hydroxyethyl starch.
iii. Metabolic acidosis results from hypotension, poor tissue perfusion and local hypoxia; this stimulates anaerobic glycolysis and excess lactic acid production. Im-proving microcirculation and tissue blood flow is most important in treating meta-bolic acidosis.
iv. The nutritional needs of the septic patient cannot be overemphasized. The im-mediate goal of nutritional support is to prevent further catabolism of the body's own nutrient stores. Enteral feeding is preferred in septic patients – disuse of the bowel pro-motes enterocyte degradation, breakdown of the blood–bowel barrier and further bac-terial translocation. In this patient, placement of a jejunostomy tube and feeding a balanced enteral formula will help restore normal metabolism.

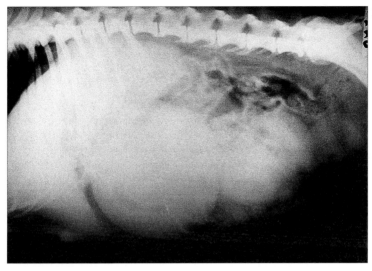

212a

212 An 11-year-old, female Fox Terrier was presented for evaluation of marked weight gain over the last three months, in spite of decreased appetite during that period of time. There were no other significant clinical signs. An abdominal radiograph of the dog is shown (212a).
i. Is the radiograph normal?
ii. What are the differential diagnoses for the noted abnormalities?
iii. What other diagnostic tools would you use before proceeding with exploratory laparotomy?

213 You are presented with a one-year-old, female Giant Schnauzer for its annual vaccinations. On auscultation of the chest you detect a murmur. Part of your diagnostic evaluation includes a selective right ventricular angiogram. The radiograph pictured demonstrates the lesion (213).
i. Name the cardiac lesion, and identify the area outlined by arrows.
ii. Describe the murmur you would hear with this type of lesion.
iii. What ECG findings would you expect with this lesion?
iv. What therapy would you recommend, and what would determine if medical or surgical therapy were indicated?

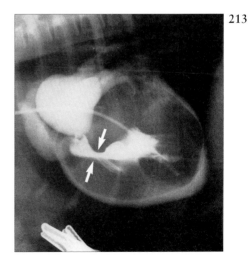

213

212b

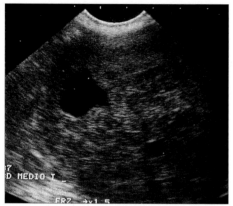

212 i. No. A large round mass (approximately 10 cm diameter) is visible in the cranial abdomen. The spleen is not visible, and a tubular structure of fluid opacity is present in the caudal abdomen, compatible with an enlarged uterus.
ii. The cranial mass could be associated with the spleen by position and because the normal shadow of the organ is not visible in this view. Differential diagnoses include a mass on the kidney, adrenal gland, mesenteric lymph node or ovary. The caudal mass is compatible with a pyometra.
iii. In this case, sonography provides data of great value. The spleen was normal in size, and the cranial mass was identified as an ovarian tumor (212b). The pyometra was readily visualized on the sonogram. The remaining abdominal organs and contralateral ovary were normal, and thoracic radiographs (three views) showed no evidence of metastases. Ovariohysterectomy was performed. Histologic evaluation of the ovary identified a papillary adenocarcinoma. This is the most common ovarian tumor type in bitches. They can spread to the lungs or seed throughout the abdomen causing carcinomatosis. Careful inspection and biopsy of suspicious lesions on the contralateral ovary and all peritoneal surfaces is warranted at the time of laparotomy. Treatment is by surgical resection. The prognosis is good if metastasis has not occurred. Chemotherapy may be effective for disseminated tumors.

213 i. Subvalvular pulmonic stenosis with muscular infundibular stenosis. The arrows outline the poststenotic dilation of the pulmonary artery.
ii. Crescendo–decrescendo systolic murmur heard best on the left side at the base of the heart.
iii. ECG changes would be consistent with right-sided cardiac enlargement and right axis deviation. Tall P waves, S waves greater than 0.35 mV in lead II and greater than 0.05 mV in lead I, presence of S waves in leads I, II, III and aVF, and deep Q waves (>0.5 mV) in leads I, II, III and aVF are consistent with right-sided cardiac enlargement.
iv. The decision between medical and surgical management of pulmonic stenosis is generally based on the pressure gradient between the right ventricle and the pulmonary artery. A catheter is placed through the right ventricle into the pulmonary artery, and pressures are monitored as the catheter is withdrawn through the stenosis. The pressure in the pulmonary artery is lower than that of the right ventricle because of obstructed flow. Surgery is recommended in adult dogs if right ventricular systolic pressure is 120 mmHg or greater (in immature dogs greater than 70 mmHg), or if the gradient across the stenosis is greater than 100 mmHg.

No specific medical therapy is indicated for the management of pulmonic stenosis. Many dogs are asymptomatic and those with clinical signs generally have pressure gradients which warrant surgery. If left untreated, signs of right-sided heart failure develop and may be managed medically.

214 With regard to the dog in **213** with pulmonic stenosis, what surgical options are available for treatment of the lesion?

215 A 14-year-old, mixed-breed dog is presented because of progressive abdominal enlargement. A positive undulation is found and paracentesis is performed. Cytologic examination of the abdominal fluid reveals reactive mesothelial cells.

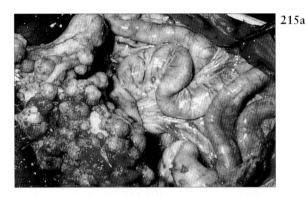

215a

i. The greater omentum (**215a**) and the abdominal wall (**215b**) are shown. What is your presumptive diagnosis?
ii. The healing of acute peritoneal defects is rapid and often complete within 5–7 days regardless of the size of the defect. Characterize this healing process.
iii. Suturing the peritoneum is not advisable. Explain why.

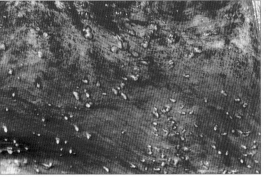

215b

216 You are planning to remove several lipomas (2–4 cm in diameter) from a healthy eight-year-old, spayed female Cocker Spaniel. The dog has moderate dental calculus and periodontitis, and the owner requests that the teeth be cleaned at the same time so that the dog will only have to undergo anesthesia once. You agree to perform both the lipoma removals and the dental cleaning/prophylaxis at the same time.
i. What potential complications should you warn the owner about?
ii. Would you use prophylactic antibiotic therapy to prevent wound infection in this dog?
iii. If you choose to use a prophylactic antibiotic, what drug would you use and when would you administer it?

214 Pulmonic stenosis with infundibular muscular stenosis carries the poorest prognosis and is the most difficult to treat surgically. Options for treating this type of stenosis are the modified Brock procedure, patch graft technique and right ventricle-pulmonary artery conduit. Techniques such as valve dilation and pulmonary arteriotomy are not successful at resolving the muscular component of this condition.

The modified Brock technique involves placing a purse-string suture and Rumel tourniquet in the right ventricle and a right ventriculotomy incision is made. An infundibular rongeur is inserted and the Rumel tightened. The subvalvular stenosis and infundibular muscle is removed. When complete, the purse-string is tied off to close the ventriculotomy. The patch graft technique involves placing a patch over the pulmonary outflow tract between the right ventricle and the pulmonary artery. A preplaced wire or cutting suture is used to cut the outflow tract, allowing blood to fill the patch and the widened outflow tract. This technique enlarges the outflow tract and allows blood to flow more easily to the pulmonary artery. The conduit technique accomplishes the same goal as the patch graft by bypassing the pulmonary outflow tract; a synthetic vascular conduit is placed between the right ventricle and the pulmonary artery. Conduits are available with or without a valve to prevent regurgitation.

215 i. Neoplastic effusion caused by a metastatic tumor, most likely a mesothelioma or gastrointestinal adenocarcinoma. Widespread peritoneal dissemination like this is also known as carcinomatosis.
ii. The healing process of the peritoneum is called reperitonealization and occurs by deposition of mesothelial cells on the denuded surface, centripetal proliferation of mesothelial cell from the wound edges, and adherence of nearby structures that have a mesothelial surface.
iii. Suturing the peritoneum is not advised because if it is left unsutured, there is less adhesion formation and no increase in dehiscence or delay in wound healing. Furthermore, suturing of the peritoneum does not increase the strength of a wound.

216 i. Potential complications of lipoma removal include hematoma, seroma, wound infection and dehiscence associated with inadvertent early removal of sutures or staples. Potential complications of dental cleaning/prophylaxis include pain or bleeding while eating and bacteremia. Common organisms associated with periodontal disease include anaerobes (*Porphyromonas* spp., *Actinomyces* spp.), streptococci and enterococci. Dental cleaning results in bacteremia, and high numbers of organisms are present in blood at the lipoma removal sites; the risk of wound infection may be higher than usual.
ii. In a healthy dog with moderate dental calculus and periodontitis, it may not be necessary to use prophylactic antibiotics. If you choose to use antibiotics to reduce the chance of wound infection, short-term perioperative use is recommended.
iii. High blood concentrations of antibiotics are required at the time blood is seeping into the surgical wound and are continued for a maximum of 24 hours. The antibiotic should be effective against the organisms prevalent in periodontal disease. The drugs of choice would be ampicillin/sulbactam (20 mg/kg, i/v, q 6 hours) or amoxicillin/clavulinic acid (11–22 mg/kg, p/o, q 8 hours). Alternative drugs would be clindamycin (11 mg/kg, p/o or i/v, q 12 hours) or tinidazole (30 mg/kg, p/o, q 24 hours, in dogs; 15 mg/kg, p/o, q 24 hours, in cats). (Tinidazole is currently available in Europe and is awaiting approval in the USA.) Intravenous drugs are administered at the time of anesthetic induction, while oral drugs are administered several hours before surgery.

217 i. Identify this instrument (217a).
ii. What is its use?
iii. What are examples of alternative instruments that can be used for the same purpose?

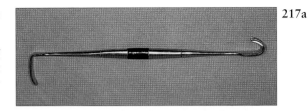

218 A lung lobectomy is being performed to remove a pulmonary abscess in the affected lobe (218a, b).
i. What instrument is being used?
ii. Describe how the device functions, and name one other application for this device.

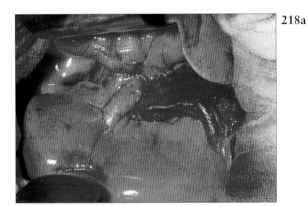

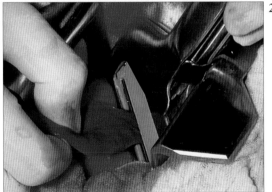

219 For what time durations do the following suture materials provide useful strength for wound closure and remain present in the surgical wound?
i. Chromic gut.
ii. Polygalactin 910 (Vicryl) or polyglycolic acid (Dexon).
iii. Polydioxanone (PDS) or polyglyconate (Maxon).
iv. Nylon.
v. Polypropylene (Prolene) or polybutester (Novafil).

217b

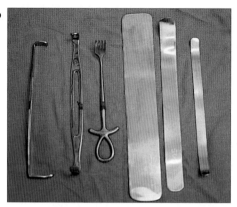

217 i. Senn retractor.
ii. To facilitate exposure and maintain retraction of adjacent or overlying tissues while the primary procedure is performed.
iii. Army-Navy, Rake, and Malleable retractors are all examples of common hand held retractors (**217b**). These instruments are an essential part of a well equipped surgical pack. They are valuable for retraction of large and small tissue, and allow a surgical field uncluttered by fingers. The main disadvantage of hand held retractors are that they require a surgical assistant. Self-retaining retractors such as Gelpi, Weitlaner and Balfour retractors maintain tissue separation without assistance.

218 i. A surgical linear stapling device. TP 90, TP 60 and TP 30 (Ethicon Endo-Surgery), and TA 90 and TA 55 (United States Surgical Corporation) are examples of linear stapling devices. The numeric designation refers to the length in millimeters of the rows of staples placed when discharged. They place a double row of staggered staples which allows circulation between the staples, assuring viability of the 2–4 mm of tissue remaining distal to the staples.
ii. Tissue to be removed is placed in the jaws of the stapler and they are closed. The adjusting knob is set to the desired amount of tissue compression. For thick and friable tissues such as liver, less compression is used to avoid cutting the tissues. The safety catch is released and the trigger is squeezed until it locks into the handle, sealing the tissue with staples. The device has a cutting guide for a scalpel to transect the tissue distal to the staples. The jaws are released and the instrument removed. The stump is inspected for leakage. The stapler allows application deep within body cavities for such procedures as resection of the right atrial appendage, pulmonary lobectomy or pneumonectomy, hepatic lobectomy, prostatic cyst resection, partial splenectomy, uterine or ovarian pedicles, and similar procedures.

219 i. 33% loss of strength at seven days; 67% loss at 28 days; complete absorption at 60 days (shorter if infection/inflammation present).
ii. Polygalactin 910: 50% loss of strength at 14 days, 80% at 21 days; complete absorption at 60–90 days. Polyglycolic acid: 37% loss of strength at seven days, 80% at 14 days; complete absorption at 120 days.
iii. Polydioxanone and polyglyconate: 19–26% loss of strength at 14 days, 41–42 % at 28 days, 86% loss at 56 days; complete absorption at 180–182 days.
iv. Biologically inert; 30% loss of strength at two years; never completely absorbed.
v. Strength is permanently retained after implantation; never absorbed.

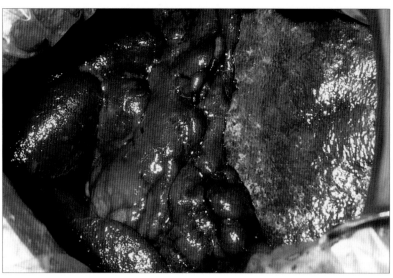

220 A five-year-old West Highland White Terrier developed jaundice, anorexia and abdominal distension one week after a dog fight. Radiographic examination of the abdomen revealed the presence of free fluid. Abdominal paracentesis revealed a dark brownish-red fluid. The exploratory laparotomy findings are shown (220).
i. What is the most likely diagnosis?
ii. Name several surgical procedures to eliminate the primary problem.
iii. What supportive therapy should be instituted?

221 A two-year-old, castrated male domestic shorthair cat is brought to your clinic after having been gone from home for a week. A 5 cm diameter open wound is present on the dorsum at the base of the tail. The wound surface is dry and there is leaf litter, gravel and dirt embedded in the surface of the wound.
i. What immediate wound care do you recommend for management of contamination and infection?
ii. What is your long-term plan for treatment of the wound?
iii. Do you administer antibiotics?

222 Describe the double valve Denver shunt, its components, functions, method for implantation and clinical applications.

220 i. Bile peritonitis secondary to extrahepatic biliary tract rupture, gall-bladder rupture, or extensive liver trauma.
ii. Primary closure or anastomosis of tears in the gall-bladder or bile ducts, closure of bile ducts over a T-tube or Y-tube, bile flow diversion techniques (cholecystoduodenostomy or cholecystojejunostomy), reimplantation of the avulsed bile duct and serosal patch grafting.
iii. Supportive therapy consists of peritoneal lavage, systemic antibiotic therapy, fluid and electrolyte replacement, and correction of any acid-base imbalance. Open abdominal drainage should be considered if there is bacterial peritonitis. Sterile bile peritonitis has a much better prognosis than bacterial contaminated bile peritonitis.

221 i. If there is a delay in wound care while you stabilize the cat, the wound is covered with a water-miscible antibiotic ointment and a sterile dressing. Once stable, the cat is anesthetized, the wound surgically prepared, and necrotic tissue and gross debris is removed. The wound is lavaged with isotonic crystalloid solution. Bacterial contamination may be further reduced with 1.0% povidone iodine solution (1 part povidone solution:10 parts crystalloid) or 0.05% chlorhexidine diacetate solution (1 part chlorhexidine diacetate solution:40 parts crystalloid). The wound is managed open under bandages that are changed 1–2 times daily for 3–5 days. The use of a wet-to-dry bandage facilitates debridement and promotes development of a viable vascular bed. The tail base is an ideal place to use a tie-over bandage.
ii. Options include second intention healing; chronic skin stretching using 'walking sutures' until delayed primary closure is achieved; a local flap; or an axial pattern flap based on the dorsal or ventral branch of the deep circumflex iliac artery.
iii. Short-term use of a systemic antibiotic will aid in reducing the bacterial contamination of wounded tissues, which speeds healing. A broad-spectrum antibiotic such as cephalexin (20 mg/kg p/o tid) is appropriate. Topical antibiotics/antiseptics can also be used although most agents delay wound healing. The clinician must weigh the risks and benefits of treating infection and delaying wound healing by applying topical substances.

222 The Denver shunt is a pleural/peritoneal-venous shunt for treatment of chronic ascites or pleural effusion. It consists of an efferent catheter, two one-way valves and an afferent catheter. The efferent catheter is placed in the abdomen or chest through a stab incision. The catheter is tunneled under the skin along the body wall to the cervical region. The pump is sutured in place over a rib so that external pressure compresses the pump diaphragm against a firm surface. The afferent catheter continues subcutaneously to the jugular vein and is inserted intravascularly to the level of the right atrium. A ligature is tied around the catheter to secure it in place and a proximal ligature is tightened to ligate the jugular permanently. With the catheter in place, fluid is pumped through the one-way valve system from the chest or abdomen into the right atrium. Denver shunts are used to treat ascites secondary to chronic protein losing enteropathy (the protein rich fluid is returned to circulation), and chylothorax (the shunt is reversed and placed so that fluid is drained from the thoracic cavity into the abdomen).

223 A nine-year-old, 30 kg German Shepherd Dog is presented for acute collapse. On physical examination, the dog is recumbent, tachypneic, tachycardic and has obvious abdominal distension. Mucous membranes are pale and dry, and capillary refill time is prolonged. Femoral pulse is weak and rapid. Abdominal radiographs show peritoneal effusion. Hemogram yields the following information: PCV 0.2 l/l (20%); serum protein 41 g/l (4.1 g/dl).
i. What type of fluid is appropriate for initial replacement therapy? At what rate of infusion? How do you monitor the animals's response to treatment?
ii. Abdominocentesis is performed and bloody fluid is obtained (PCV 0.14 l/l (14%); protein 38 g/l (3.8 g/dl)), confirming the presence of intraperitoneal hemorrhage. What criteria are used to decide if a transfusion is needed? What type of blood product (whole blood, packed red cells, plasma, etc.), and volume would you infuse?
iii. Despite aggressive fluid therapy and blood transfusion, the animal's condition deteriorates. Exploratory laparotomy is performed and a hemorrhaging mass is found in the spleen. A liter of blood is removed from the abdominal cavity. Do you utilize this fluid to autotransfuse this patient, or continue with whole blood transfusions?

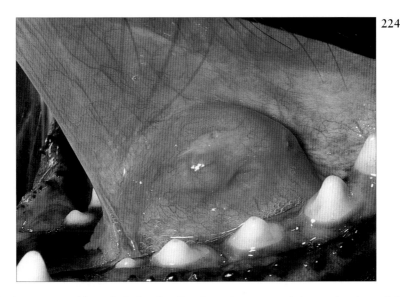

224

224 A ten-year-old, male Labrador Retriever is presented for evaluation of this tongue mass (224). The owners report no associated clinical signs; the lesion was noted incidentally when the dog was panting.
i. What are the differential diagnoses?
ii. What further tests are indicated?
iii. What is the treatment for this abnormality?

223, 224: Answers

223 i. Crystalloid agents are adequate to restore circulating volume initially. An ideal replacement solution is sodium-based, isoosmolar (canine normal 290–310 mOsm/l), has a physiologically balanced electrolyte composition, and a bicarbonate precursor such as lactate. Lactated Ringer's solution closely matches these characteristics. The rate for fluid restoration in circulatory shock is 90 ml/kg/hour for dogs and 60 ml/kg/hour for cats. Hypertonic saline (7.5%) and colloids such as hydroxyethyl starch (Hetastarch, Dupont Critical Care) and dextran 70 (Gentran 70, Baxter Health Care) increase intravascular volume by raising serum osmolarity and activating fluid shifts from the interstitium to the vascular space (canine dose – 4-8 ml/kg for 7.5% saline and 20 ml/kg for colloids). Use of an osmotic agent decreases the volume of crystalloid solution required to restore perfusion. Restoration of intravascular volume is recognized by normalization of heart rate, respiratory rate, pulse quality, mucous membrane color and capillary refill time.
ii. Animals require red cell replacement for acute hemorrhage when 25–30% of blood volume is lost (blood volume in this dog is 90 ml/kg, i.e. 2700 ml), when PCV declines acutely below 0.2 l/l (20%) and when clinical signs indicate cardiovascular function is compromised. Packed red blood cells with crystalloid fluids, or whole blood are best administered; whole blood has the advantage of replacing clotting factors. Red cells are administered to maintain PCV above 0.15 l/l (15%); a guideline of 10–20 ml of blood/kg body weight or one unit of blood (500 ml) per 20 kg animal can be used.
iii. Autotransfusion is contraindicated due to the likelihood of spreading or seeding tumor cells system wide. Use of whole blood transfusions is preferred for this patient. Ideally, cross-match is performed prior to all transfusions; here the need for multiple transfusions requires it.

224 i. The most common canine tongue neoplasm is squamous cell carcinoma. Other common tumor types are granular cell myoblastoma, melanoma and mast cell tumor. Sarcomas occur less commonly, and a variety of other carcinomas and benign tumors have occasionally been reported.
ii. The tongue is biopsied by wedge excision from the center of the mass. The surgeon must be careful not to extend the tumor margin at the time of biopsy. Regional lymph nodes are aspirated to stage the tumor, and if melanoma or squamous cell carcinoma is suspected, thoracic radiographs are performed (left and right lateral, and ventrodorsal views) to search for metastasis.
iii. Surgical excision is the treatment of choice for most lingual tumors. Granular cell myoblastoma is potentially a curable tumor with wide surgical excision, and good local control (65%) can be achieved with melanoma. Long-term survival (>18 months) often occurs with lingual melanomas as metastases seem to occur more slowly than for melanomas at other sites. Squamous cell carcinoma and mast cell tumor have a poor prognosis for one year survival (25% or less); local recurrence and lymph node metastases are common. In general, tumors of the rostral tongue have a better prognosis. Adjuvant chemotherapy and radiation are recommended for inoperable tumors, when lymph node metastases are present or likely to occur (melanoma, squamous cell carcinoma, mast cell tumor), to shrink tumors before surgery, and to manage metastases.

225 This ten-year-old Golden Retriever (225) had a history of weakness, restlessness, exercise intolerance, seizures and collapse. Hypoglycemia was found by serial measurements of plasma glucose.
i. What is the diagnosis?
ii. Name two other primary pancreatic neoplasms.
iii. Give the prognosis for this dog after surgery and discuss some prognostic factors.

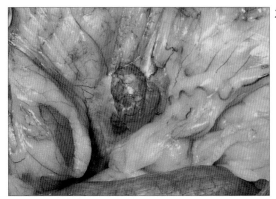

225

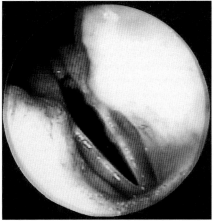

226a

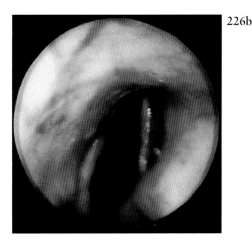

226b

226 This is an intraoral endoscopic picture of an eight-year-old, spayed female Labrador Retriever that presented to the emergency clinic for dyspnea (226a). The owners reported an acute onset of respiratory distress; upon further questioning, you learn that the dog has also had a change in her bark and she seemed to have respiratory difficulties last summer as well.
i. Based on the history and illustration, what is your preliminary diagnosis?
ii. How will you confirm the diagnosis?
iii. Name three surgical procedures that can be used to correct this problem and what complications might be encountered with each? A postoperative intraoral endoscopic view of this animal is shown (226b).

225 i. Insulin-secreting islet cell neoplasm (insulinoma). Diagnosis is confirmed by measuring a high serum insulin concentration concurrent with a low blood glucose (see 17).
ii. Exocrine pancreatic adenocarcinoma and gastrinoma.
iii. The short-term prognosis is very good for relief of signs of hypoglycemia, however the long-term prognosis is generally poor because a surgical cure is unlikely given the highly metastic behavior of the tumor. Relapse of clinical signs can be expected 10–14 months after surgery in about 95% of the cases. Poor prognostic indicators include age at time of diagnosis, high preoperative insulin concentrations and the presence of distant metastases at time of surgery.

226 i. Laryngeal paralysis. Idiopathic laryngeal paralysis is usually seen in large-breed dogs (Retrievers, Saint Bernard, and Siberian Husky) over nine years of age. Other etiologies include trauma, hypothyroidism and congenital paralysis. Clinical signs include voice change; gagging or coughing while eating; inspiratory stridor; and dyspnea, cyanosis or even syncope.
ii. Diagnosis is by laryngoscopic observation of the arytenoids under sedation light enough that the gag reflex remains present. Failure of the arytenoid cartilages to abduct during inspiration or cough is diagnostic. Cervical and thoracic radiographs are made to rule out other possible respiratory diseases.
iii. Three surgical procedures are:

• Unilateral arytenoid lateralization. Variations of this procedure include thyro-arytenoid and cricoarytenoid cartilage lateralization. The most common complications are aspiration pneumonia and postoperative edema or hematoma. It is possible to penetrate the laryngeal mucosa during dissection, contaminating the surgical field from the oral cavity and risking abscess formation at the surgical site. In this author's opinion (N.J.H. Sharp), this technique is the treatment of choice.
• Partial laryngectomy is performed *per os* after temporary tracheostomy intubation (this allows unencumbered visualization of the pharynx). Hemorrhage and subsequent aspiration of blood can occur with this procedure, and swelling and edema may lead to airway obstruction. Aspiration pneumonia can occur if too much of the larynx is excised and the epiglottis is incapable of covering the airway. The most severe complication is laryngeal webbing and stenosis weeks to months after surgery.
• Castellated laryngofissure widens the lumen of the glottis by apposition of a stair-stepped incision in the thyroid cartilage. The vocal folds are also resected and mattress sutures are placed through the arytenoid and thyroid cartilages to stabilize the arytenoid cartilages. Tracheostomy is recommended prior to this procedure. Complications reported include edema, aspiration pneumonia and stenosis at the surgery site.

227 Name three disinfectants used for preparation of the surgical field. List the mechanism of action, advantages and disadvantages of each.

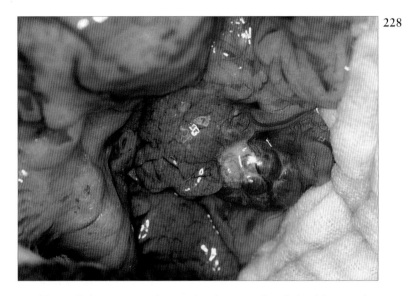

228 An additional diagnostic technique has been used to help delineate this tumor during surgery (228).
i. Name this technique.
ii. What deleterious side-effects can occur from an excessive dose?
iii. Name another type of tumor in which this technique is helpful.

229 A three-year-old, castrated male domestic shorthair cat is presented for emergency evaluation after being hit by a car. Prior to the accident the cat was normal. Outwardly, the cat appears normal on clinical examination except for a heart rate of 185 bpm and a respiratory rate of 55 breaths per minute.
i. What type of 'occult' injuries can be present that may not be readily apparent on routine physical examination?
ii. You are concerned the cat may have a ruptured bladder. How will you assess this further?
iii. What is the treatment for a ruptured bladder?

227 Chlorhexidine alters bacterial cell wall permeability causing precipitation of cellular proteins and cell death. Advantages include rapid onset of action (99% kill rate within 30 seconds), broad spectrum of activity (most bacteria and many fungi), prolonged residual activity, and continued activity in the presence of organic matter and alcohol. Disadvantages include decreased efficacy against some *Pseudomonas* spp., minimal viricidal and sporicidal activity, and, rarely, contact dermatitis.

Povidone slowly releases free iodine which binds to bacterial cell walls creating free radicals that result in cell death. Advantages include rapid onset of action (similar to chlorhexidine) and broad spectrum of activity (most bacteria, any viruses, fungi, some protozoa, and sporicidal after prolonged exposure). Disadvantages include inactivation in the presence of organic matter, minimal residual activity, skin irritation and staining.

Isopropyl alcohol reacts with lipids in bacterial cell membranes leading to altered permeability and cell death. Advantages include broad spectrum of activity, rapid onset, ability to remove the detergent left by other agents (e.g. chlorhexidine scrub, povidone scrub) and increased efficacy of chlorhexidine and povidone when used with alcohol. Disadvantages include slower onset of action and less efficacy than chlorhexidine or povidone iodine when used alone, little residual activity, and tissue injury and necrosis in open wounds.

228 i. Methylene blue (3 mg/kg body weight) can be given intravenously to delineate insulinomas and their metastases. Methylene blue appears to stain specifically the pancreatic islet-cell tumor cells, facilitating visualization of small masses at surgery.
ii. Side-effects include pseudocyanosis, hemolytic anemia with Heinz body formation and red blood cell morphology changes, disseminated intravascular coagulation and hemoglobinephrosis.
iii. Parathyroid gland tumors.

229 i. Occult thoracic injuries from trauma include pneumothorax, pulmonary contusion, diaphragmatic hernia (especially in cats) and rib fractures. Occult abdominal injuries include splenic and hepatic contusion or laceration, biliary tract rupture, and urinary tract injury or rupture.
ii. Four-quadrant abdominocentesis is performed and recovered fluid is grossly inspected and evaluated for PCV, protein content, cytology and urea nitrogen. Comparison is made with systemic PCV, serum protein concentration and serum urea nitrogen. High concentrations of urea nitrogen and the presence of significant amounts of blood in abdominal fluid indicates urinary tract rupture. If urine is identified in the abdomen, the animal is further evaluated by excretory urogram and contrast cystourethrogram to assess the integrity of the kidneys, ureters, bladder and urethra, and identify the location of leakage before surgery.
iii. If the animal is not immediately stable for surgery, a peritoneal and urinary catheter are placed to drain urine from the abdomen and bladder. Fluids and other medications are administered to stabilize and diurese the animal. Surgical repair is performed when the patient is stable and azotemia is decreased; in some cases this may be 24–72 hours after presentation. A caudal ventral midline laparotomy is made and the urinary tract is inspected for signs of injury. The bladder rent is debrided as necessary and sutured with a single or double layer closure using absorbable suture. If the rent is large or bladder wall integrity is questionable, a urinary catheter is left in place for several days after surgery.

Index

tissue
  adhesives 63, 127
  expander 87, 88
  flaps 2
tongue squamous cell carcinoma 224
tonsillar squamous cell carcinoma 69
tooth extraction 138
trachea
  avulsion 13
  hypoplasia 34
tracheal collapse 156
tracheal laceration 103
tracheal resection and anastomosis 156
tracheal ring prostheses 156
trachealis muscle plication 156
tracheostomy, temporary 34
transfusion 223
trauma 78
  chest 54
  degloving 123, 162
  diaphragmatic hernia 196, 197
  inguinal region 149
  occult injuries 229
  open wound 101
  renal 151
  renal/ureteral injury 96
  ruptured bladder 229
  tracheal laceration 103
Trichuris worm 90
tube thoracostomy 155
tubular adenocarcinoma 104
tumor
  of dental origin 116, 179
  staging 19, 44, 55, 69, 116
  thrombus 118, 119
typhlectomy 90

umbilical hernia 4
upper airway obstruction 208
urachal diverticulum 130, 131
urachus, persistent 130
ureteral ectopia 91, 114
ureterocele 35
ureterocolonic anastomosis 183
ureterotomy 14
urethral obstruction 67, 106
  urachal diverticulum 131
urethral prolapse 110
urethral stricture 166
urethral tear 151
urethrorectal fistula, congenital 172

urethrostomy 45
  perineal 49
  prepubic 166
urethrotomy, prescrotal 45
urinary bladder
  ruptured 229
  transitional cell carcinoma 183
urinary calculi 133
urinary drainage system, indwelling 67
urinary obstruction 49
urinary tract infection 36, 50, 130
  urethral stricture 166
urolith 56, 80, 59
urolithiasis 14, 59
uroretroperitoneum 96
uterine neoplasia 161
uterus, fluid-filled 18

vaginal hyperplasia 159, 160
vaginal neoplasia 159
vaginal prolapse 159, 160
vaginal stricture 180
vaginography 180
vaginoplasty 180
Van Langenbeck technique 53
vascular clamp 23
vascular ligation 192
vascular ring anomaly 191
venotomy 23
ventricular pacemaker implantation 42
vesica duplex 187
vesicourachal diverticulum, congenital 130
vincristine 117
volvulus, mesenteric 9
vomiting 33, 109
Von Willebrand's disease 150

Whipple's triad 17
wound
  contraction 65
  dehiscence 95
  infection 10
wound closure
  soft tissue sarcoma resection 111
  trauma 149
wound healing
  burns 199
  second intention 123
  stages 31

Z-plasty 65
Zepp procedure, modified 129